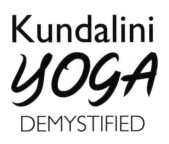

Kundalini
YOGA
DEMYSTIFIED

About the Author

Erin Elizabeth Downing (she/her) recovered from debilitating illness and food allergies with the help of Eastern healing modalities. Today she is a certified Kundalini yoga and Pilates instructor, holding certificates in wellness coaching and plant-based nutrition. She is a sought-after coach and speaker, bringing her philosophy of paying yourself first—mind, body, and spirit—to her clients and events.

To Write to the Author

If you wish to contact the author or would like more information about this book, please write to the author in care of Llewellyn Worldwide Ltd. and we will forward your request. Both the author and publisher appreciate hearing from you and learning of your enjoyment of this book and how it has helped you. Llewellyn Worldwide Ltd. cannot guarantee that every letter written to the author can be answered, but all will be forwarded. Please write to:

Erin Elizabeth Downing
℅ Llewellyn Worldwide
2143 Wooddale Drive
Woodbury, MN 55125-2989
Please enclose a self-addressed stamped envelope for reply,
or $1.00 to cover costs. If outside the U.S.A., enclose
an international postal reply coupon.

Many of Llewellyn's authors have websites with additional information and resources. For more information, please visit our website at http://www.llewellyn.com.

ERIN ELIZABETH DOWNING

Kundalini *YOGA* DEMYSTIFIED

A Modern Guide to What It Is and How to Practice

Llewellyn Publications
Woodbury, Minnesota

First Edition
First Printing, 2021

Book design by Samantha Peterson
Cover design by Kevin R. Brown
Interior illustrations by Julia Marina Massimino
Interior illustrations on pages 54–61 by Llewellyn Art Department

All Kundalini yoga kriyas, meditations, and concepts from Kundalini Yoga as taught by Yogi Bhajan® are used courtesy of the Kundalini Research Institute. ALL RIGHTS RESERVED. Reprinted with permission. To request permission for any such items, please write to the KRI at PO Box 1819, Santa Cruz, New Mexico, 87567 or visit www.kundaliniresearchinstitute.org.

Llewellyn is a registered trademark of Llewellyn Worldwide Ltd.

Library of Congress Cataloging-in-Publication Data
Names: Downing, Erin Elizabeth, author.
Title: Kundalini yoga demystified : a modern guide to what it is and how to
    practice / by Erin Elizabeth Downing.
Description: First edition. | Woodbury, MN : Llewellyn Worldwide, [2021] |
    Includes bibliographical references. | Summary: "This book is designed
    to help the reader find balance, increase strength, and begin or
    embolden their own personal Kundalini practice" —Provided by publisher.
Identifiers: LCCN 2021027540 (print) | LCCN 2021027541 (ebook) | ISBN
    9780738767475 (paperback) | ISBN 9780738767734 (ebook)
Subjects: LCSH: Kundalini.
Classification: LCC BL1238.56.K86 D69 2021 (print) | LCC BL1238.56.K86
    (ebook) | DDC 204/.36—dc23
LC record available at https://lccn.loc.gov/2021027540
LC ebook record available at https://lccn.loc.gov/2021027541

Llewellyn Worldwide Ltd. does not participate in, endorse, or have any authority or responsibility concerning private business transactions between our authors and the public.
    All mail addressed to the author is forwarded, but the publisher cannot, unless specifically instructed by the author, give out an address or phone number.
    Any internet references contained in this work are current at publication time, but the publisher cannot guarantee that a specific location will continue to be maintained. Please refer to the publisher's website for links to authors' websites and other sources.

Llewellyn Publications
A Division of Llewellyn Worldwide Ltd.
2143 Wooddale Drive
Woodbury, MN 55125-2989
www.llewellyn.com

Printed in the United States of America

For Momma…

Momma,
You were always the light, paving the way through the darkness
The grace in my stance and the gumption behind my convictions
Now, I see you, as the wind beneath my wings
The angel ever valiantly fighting by my side
My companion in the silent battles that only my heart can see
You always loved me in my entirety
The one who saw my strengths and weaknesses
Celebrating the duality and complexity of both
Ensuring the love from your heart was always my lighthouse home
I love you, Momma
This dream fulfilled is dedicated to you
Dedicated to the sacrifices you made each day so that I might thrive
Dedicated to the tenacity in which you loved me
And to the loyalty with which you honored your friends
You were an angel in life and now in death
I pray this work makes you proud
I pray that it aids in putting your soul at ease
The knowledge that its contents will help so many
And that it was your heart that paved the way
The way for your daughter's love to pour so freely to others
Gratitude will never be enough to encompass this moment
I love you, Momma
More than all of the stars in the sky
Rest in peace knowing that I still feel your warmth and love
Each and every day
Rest knowing that you will forever be my lighthouse
And through my life, the light that is you will always shine

The work within is not my own.

The dialogue that follows represents my intuitive interpretation of these teachings and how to apply the techniques in modern life, but to be clear, this did not begin with me.

These lessons and teachings have been passed down through millennia; there have been generations of practitioners honoring and evolving this medicine with the ebb and flow of life. I express my sincere gratitude to my teachers and those who have dedicated their lives to this work. Without their wisdom and openness to share these ancient traditions, I would not be capable of sharing their knowledge with you.

The lineages on which Kundalini was founded, the texts and traditions in which these teachings reside, deserve respect. I am but a vessel, humbly translating these traditions with the prayer that they may serve. Serve the highest and best for all. Serve across all religions, races, and cultures; across socioeconomic status, sexual orientation, geography, and gender.

Again, I would like to reiterate that this book contains my interpretations of these exercises, techniques, philosophies, and practices. The words within are but a jumping-off point to begin a lifelong journey inward, tools that will help us do as Kundalini intends—bring us home to ourselves.

Contents

Exercise List[*]

* Denotes Kundalini yoga teachings as taught by Yogi Bhajan.

Disclaimer

The information in this book is not meant to diagnose, treat, prescribe, or substitute consultation with a licensed healthcare professional. If you are experiencing any medical conditions or are unsure if a pose or exercise is safe for you, consult your doctor. The techniques in this book are not recommended for children. Some yoga postures and techniques are not advised for adults who are pregnant or have just given birth.

Consult a licensed physician before beginning any new exercise or dietary regimen, especially if you have existing or potential medical conditions, and inform your physician of any nutritional changes.

Both the author and the publisher recommend that you consult a medical practitioner before attempting the techniques outlined in this book and waive all responsibility for possible consequences, including, but not limited to, injuries incurred while practicing the book's postures, techniques, and exercises. Practice at your own risk.

Foreword

ERIN ELIZABETH DOWNING IS a gift. I had the grace of meeting her in person through the synchronistic webs of the global yoga communities we are part of. When I encountered her, I felt that familiar presence that is uncommon in our world—clarity, grace, tenacity, here-ness, peace, and tenderness. I also encountered a soul who emanated the fragrance of loving kindness. That type of presence is born of deep practice of the techniques she will show you in this book. For that presence to become deep, sustained, stable, genuine, and authentic, the essence of these teachings must be brought into every area of life—especially the places that hurt and scare us. Erin has done that impeccably. As a result, she is a qualified and potent guide in your own journey of coming home to yourself. Her book will give you a compass so that you can gracefully and powerfully read the coordinates of your life and connect to your destiny.

Erin's book is not just a manual for health and awakening. While it is certainly a wise and powerful manual, it is really a deeply personal memoir of awakening that is a potent medicine for the times. While Erin spent meaningful time formally learning her art and craft in India, her essential journey of awakening has been the deep, gritty, and powerful love story of a soul waking up to itself. Wherever we are in this world, there is an inner home, a sacred sanctuary, that is our original space and safest shelter. These practices, honed through thousands of years of refinement, help us come into that space. While we cannot study the invisible worlds of energy and prana easily, we can study the effects of yoga, and as we progress in our modern world, the findings are unequivocal: Breath, meditation, and yoga are really, really, really good for you on just about every level of human existence.

I began my journey with meditation thirty-five years ago and have never turned back. Yogic practice and meditation empowered me to rise above very challenging and traumatic circumstances that I faced as a young boy. I have spent three and a half decades of my life studying, practicing, and learning the art and science of mind-body health care. I have met and studied with living masters from several traditions, Eastern and Western. I have personally witnessed truly supernatural feats by living masters of the East. As a busy health care provider, I have devoted my life to helping people heal from the damage of stress, providing ways to live healthier, happier, and fuller lives. There is no doubt in my mind that yoga, in its essence, is one of the most powerful medicines we have access to.

Movement, awareness, and breath are three simple but extraordinarily powerful tools that level up and heal the body's stress response, improve brain function, enhance immune system balance, improve cardiovascular function, restore healthy metabolism, and even improve the capacity to think, be empathic, and take meaningful action in life. If we could bottle what is in this book and sell it as a pill, it would be a trillion dollar drug. Thankfully, however, it is not. The beauty of Erin's book is not in the incredible results you will likely achieve if you practice patiently, persistently, and diligently, the miracle of this book is who you will become in the process. I love this book because in each sentence you can feel both Erin's deep, embodied love pouring through while simultaneously feeling the ancient, luminous, and powerful teachings that come from the Kundalini lineage of yoga. The book is a crucible that can literally birth your calling. It can serve as a biodome in which you can re-create the ecosystem of your life in joyful and healing ways.

In health care, I spent countless hours learning about "evidence-based" medicine. Ironically, however, the vast majority of all new research that comes out is based on pathogenesis. Literally, this word means the origin of a disease. Attention is focused almost entirely on what went wrong and how to fix it. This has been extremely useful over the last century and a half, as health care practitioners have done amazing things to alleviate suffering in human beings. However, there is a paltry amount of research spent on salutogenesis, or the origin of health. This scientific framework gives us perspectives and tools to discover what creates life, health, healing, and well-being. Salutogenesis is just as important as pathogenesis. In the latter, we learn the science-based tools that help us live in potent harmony and coherence with our own self-healing and self-regulatory potential. In industrialized society, where the majority of the most deadly diseases are stress related (mental, emotional, dietary, and structural stress), this is no longer a luxury. It is a radical necessity. As the milieu of the microbiome and holobiome are radically broken down by sedentary lifestyles, processed foods, and an increasing level of stress brought on by mass media and social media, this book is a clear stream of light that illuminates the void many people feel.

In our society, however, it is easy to become cynical of anything that, at first glance, does not pass the reductionist and materialist worldview that only what can be seen, touched, and physically measured is real. This pervasive view often keeps people who would greatly benefit from these practices from participating in them. While more research is deeply needed as we explore the terrain of mind, body, and spirit in health care, this book demystifies the mystical. That is a gift of this book. That is no small thing; it gets us out of our chairs and onto the mat to do the joyful work of yoga. It is only through intentional action that we transform ourselves and this world. And as yoga, meditation, the breath, and chakras are looked at from a scientific altitude, it radically empowers us to practice. This attitude takes nothing from ancient wisdom; it gives it more texture, flavor, and wonder.

Without practice, this book is simply more philosophy. If you will lovingly and courageously engage with it, taking it at your own pace, it will serve as an initiation into your most glorious life. After many sessions of practice (especially when you may not feel like it) you will in fact greet your true self. You will come home. You will be a living temple of wisdom, vitality, kindness, and grit.

May Erin's book inspire you, guide you, and become one of your compasses that you keep with you in your handbag, in your car, and dog-eared and underlined by your bed. I assure you, diligent and playful practice will not dull any part of you. Rather, it will awaken a radiant and effervescent fullness of life. You will learn to be fully yourself. It will relax your brow and bring a smile to your face. It will awaken within you a mighty kindness.

Dr. Matt lyon

Introduction

THIS IS A BOOK about Kundalini yoga, an ancient yoga lineage that, until now, has gotten a bit of a bad rap. Toted as "hippie" or "woowoo," Kundalini yoga has a reputation of being too far out there to be easily digested by the masses. In this book, we are embarking on a journey to change that. Kundalini yoga is a unique form of magic, yes, but that does not mean it is unattainable. Anything new is something unfamiliar. Unfamiliar does not mean good, threatening, or anything in between. It merely means unknown. Every time you step into the unknown, it is a leap of faith—a leap made all that much easier with a trusted friend by your side. Down the rabbit hole of Kundalini, I am excited to be that friend, accompanying you on this journey, quelling your fears, and encouraging you every step of the way.

Within, you will find a glossary with easy-to-understand definitions and an appendix that makes quickly finding exercises a breeze. The exercises are organized based on the amount of time you have to practice. Whether it be one, three, or eleven minutes, there is a way to squeeze in your Kundalini yoga practice, and this book will show you how. At the end of each chapter, detailed techniques allow you to immediately place what you have learned into action. Kundalini is a practice rooted in yogic science and we capitalize on that science by wasting no time, so you will find easy-to-perform exercises in chapter 1. The short chapter lengths combined with the follow-up practices make learning the foundations of Kundalini an intuitive journey. By taking the process one step—or chapter—at a time, you remain in the driver's seat, dictating the cadence as you go.

Each chapter is a by-product of the knowledge I gained during my time studying Kundalini and Ayurvedic nutrition in India. The cadence of my education introduced a multitude of topics at once. Unlike this book, the tempo of my journey was not under my control. Both physically and mentally rigorous, the days were master planned from sunup to sundown. It is a sign of intelligence to hold two opposing ideas within the mind simultaneously, but keeping five to ten *new* ideas at the forefront of consciousness overloads the circuiting.[1] Though my Kundalini teacher training was a life-altering experience, the intensity of that training heavily influenced the starkly different approach found within. This book is a culmination of my knowledge of Kundalini yoga, creating a unique blend of traditions and exercises.

This book comes nowhere near the level of continuous mental agility that I experienced while studying to be a Kundalini yoga teacher. Dedicating one's life to the pursuit of an endeavor is what makes that level of intense study attainable. Even with years of Kundalini yoga practice under my belt, I found my mental fortitude stretched to its limit. Reading this book is not your sole purpose, nor should it be, and it is with that in mind that the content is structured. If you are familiar with some of the topics, you might fly through a chapter or two. If you aren't, it may take a week, two, three, or ten to deeply digest and incorporate the material. The keyword here is *incorporate*.

One of the things that makes Kundalini life-altering is the compounding effect of its nature. I was taught that the results of practicing Kundalini for just three minutes every day far outweigh the results of a ninety-minute class once a week. Within you will come to understand the yogic science behind this claim as well as many others, gaining not only knowledge but personal licensing to make your Kundalini practice your own. The thing that drew me to yoga over sixteen years ago was the revelation that it was different every time I stepped onto my mat.

Instructors lay the foundation, provide you with tools, and create a roadmap to follow. This book is intentionally structured so that the foundation of all yoga lineages, as a science and a practice, are introduced in the opening chapters, not only the teachings of the lineage of Kundalini. Taught in this way, you first learn why yogis do what they do. This is purposely explained to bridge the connections between the natural world and the spiritual. In this book, you won't find pretty pictures demonstrating gravity-defying yoga postures. What you will find is an in-depth knowledge of yoga, its history, information about how and why Kundalini is performed, and what results are waiting for you on the other side.

---

1. Fitzgerald, "The Crack-Up."

How to Use This Book

Even if you have prior experience with Kundalini, reading these pages with an open mind will awaken your body in life-altering ways. Asking you to show up with a clear heart and mind is a big ask. It is one I do not take lightly, and one I have thought through with extreme care. There is no wrong way to move through these pages, whether you spend a year practicing one chapter or fly through the entire book in one weekend. I think of books as living, breathing entities. Each holds a unique heartbeat and personalized instruction for the reader it calls home. Therefore, I encourage you to highlight to your heart's content. Dog-ear, underline, scribble notes, write poems, and insert modifications as you feel called. Don't worry about the book being too pretty to mess up. As they say in the movie *Letters to Juliet*, "Life *is* the messy bits." Scribble, scrabble, and make this guide your own.

Journal as you read. Take notes on your phone, on your computer, or in a notebook, or talk it through with a friend. Joining a book club or finding a spiritual running buddy is a beautiful way to not only hold yourself accountable but to build a community of like-minded individuals. Not everyone has to think as you do to receive your love, but having a soul friend who understands your journey is an invaluable gift. A trusted health-care provider is another invaluable tool to aid in this process. Emotions will likely come up that need to be healed, and speaking to a therapist, friend, or doctor can make these transitions more manageable.

Regardless of your prior experience with Kundalini, I suggest picking one exercise and sticking with it. Don't let the magnitude of activities within this book bog you down. Pick one and commit to doing it every day for the next seven days. Then commit to extending your practice through the end of the month. Keep reading the chapters as you desire, but stick to one exercise until it becomes second nature. You will have plenty of time to work through each activity, but choosing and maintaining one practice will make all the difference. Should you get a wild hair and want to try new exercises in addition to the first, excellent! Do one in the morning and one at night. Discipline does not mean there is no room for flexibility. Add other techniques in and out as you choose while practicing the first exercise on repeat.

As you proceed, I suggest you move through this book as written. The most seasoned yogis may find the foundational information a quick review potentially worth skipping over, but I promise there is a nugget of guidance your soul is begging to hear. Be it part of your everyday repertoire or something new and unknown; you are set up for success by starting at the beginning. This is not just a book about Kundalini yoga as a medium for change. Each chapter builds on the one before. By focusing on the practice's foundations first, we create solid ground for knowledge to flourish.

The Chapters Ahead

In the pages that follow, you will find a progression of chapters explaining what Kundalini is. In chapter 1, you will discover an overview of Kundalini's techniques and definitions. Here you will find foundational knowledge of Kundalini, what makes it different from other yoga lineages, and how Kundalini came to the Western world. A condensed glossary of Kundalini's most utilized terms provides a foundational understanding. Kundalini's frequently asked questions are answered in chapter 1.

In chapter 2, we discuss the routines of a yogi so that you learn how to implement them in your life. You will learn how to utilize Mother Nature's wisdom to rise with the sun and create new habits with the seasons' change. Terms such as *ambrosia hours* are defined, and theories such as why you should use a yoga mat are explained.

In chapter 3, we dive deep into the wisdom of the chakras. I introduce each chakra in detail and explain the order in which we move through them to unlock and ignite Kundalini energy.

In chapter 4, we discuss balancing the masculine and feminine energies within each of us. You are introduced to the three most important nadis and will come to understand how to utilize their power to bring balance and harmony into your body. Here you will also get an in-depth introduction to your Kundalini energy, where it resides, and why you should strive to awaken it.

In chapter 5, we discuss the nutritional wisdom of the yogis to detoxify and strengthen the body. You will learn why cows are sacred in India while discovering the yogic philosophy behind fasting and eating with the seasons. You will come to understand the importance of your digestive fire and how to support your body during a Kundalini awakening.

In chapter 6, your Kundalini yoga practice's most-utilized postures are introduced. You will receive instructions to set a solid foundation for your practice, learn why alignment is so important, and find detailed explanations for why things are done in the order prescribed.

In chapter 7, your Kundalini practice's foundational breathing techniques are explained. You will use pranayama breathwork to detoxify your body, utilizing the postures and alignment learned in the chapter before. By understanding the five prana divisions, you will learn how your body uses this life force energy to expel waste and operate at maximum capacity. Learning how to use the breath to maximize your body's potential will change how you utilize your lungs to amplify your Kundalini practice going forward.

Chapter 8 will instruct how to utilize the power of mudras to direct the intention of your practice and create lasting change. You will understand the different types of mudras and how to use them to unlock the power of the planets and elements.

In chapter 9, we demystify the magic of bandhas. Here you will come to utilize multiple prior techniques in combination with new intrinsic muscle constrictions to move past blockages within the body. The body's psychic knots are explained, and the theories on why their untying is so important are discussed.

In chapter 10, the vibrations of mantras are utilized to amplify your practice's intentions out into the world. Here you will use the power of OM and the other seed mantras to activate the energy center of the chakras.

Chapter 11 introduces the more in-depth techniques of kriyas to string together exercises that amplify your practice's intention. The previous chapters' techniques combine to create the desired result, tying together the culmination of your Kundalini journey.

Each chapter's lessons are followed by methods to help you strengthen your learning. The exercises put the yogic wisdom just explained into practice before moving forward to the next method or chapter.

Why Me?

My journey to health and wellness has been a windy one. In my early twenties I was hospitalized, debilitated by physical ailments. The ability to move through life with ease, void of pain and discomfort, was a dream deemed unattainable. One autoimmune diagnosis later (and after many failed solutions via modern Western medicine), I started down a path to educate myself on holistic and alternative healing techniques. Over the last fifteen years I have traveled the world studying modalities at their source, learning from those who have dedicated their lives to these techniques.

The day I removed meat from my diet, my quality of life improved 70 percent. As a kid who ate only lettuce and tomato on a bun in lieu of the hamburgers devoured by her peers, from a young age I understood that meat did not agree with my body. Society told me I needed meat for protein, and for years I blindly followed the words of others and ignored my body's intuition, becoming sicker with each passing year. The immediate improvement in my ailments after removing meat was my first lesson in learning to trust my gut. Diving headfirst, as I tend to do, once I recognized the healing power of a plant-based lifestyle, I devoured every book and lecture in sight, eventually obtaining a certificate in plant-based nutrition from Cornell University.

As the years progressed and my stress increased, new ailments surfaced. My stressed-out life as a New Yorker was wreaking havoc on my health. A plethora of new healers later, I was diagnosed with autoimmune diseases two and three. I double and tripled down on learning in my free time, using every vacation day to travel across the globe and experience modalities firsthand. Though I found immense relief in the methods I discovered, it was Kundalini that finally awakened the mind-body connection I had been missing. With the power of Kundalini, I discovered the connection between my brain and my gut, heightened my intuition, and began to transform from the inside out.

Through the power of Kundalini, I became a new person. My high-power, predominantly male executive colleagues began to ask what I was doing, noticing a change in my demeanor, attitude, and overall approach to my work. When I told them I discovered Kundalini, they asked me if there was a place I could direct them to learn more. Unfortunately, at the time, the answer was always no. I joked that I should post a few videos demonstrating how to practice, followed by a resounding, "Yes! Please do!" and "As soon as you do, let me know!" I rolled my eyes and laughed, but the seed had been planted. In the back of my mind, I wondered just how far this Kundalini journey would challenge me to go.

Eventually, my internal landscape changed so drastically that I outgrew my old life. Now a square peg attempting to fit into a round hole, the view from midtown Manhattan no longer felt like home. The Universe pushed me off the proverbial cliff, and a month after leaving my old life behind, I found myself on a plane to India to study Kundalini at the source. I spent the next few months researching, writing, and traveling the world, continuing down my evolutional journey with every plane, train, boat, bus, automobile, and page written. This book was created in seven countries and eighteen cities, just before (and during) a global pandemic.

To say that the content within changed drastically during this time would be an understatement. As people of every race, religion, country, ethnicity, and gender have been forced into isolation, the acceleration of the global consciousness has continued to grow. Out of great heartache and sorrow come the sweetest rewards, and as the divides between rich and poor, left and right, black and white, and gay and straight and every identifier in between continue to be pushed in opposition, I have hope. Hope because I know that the hearts of so many have been cracked open, the veil of what people "should" do fades to reveal what we are *meant* to. I see in the lives of so many others an awakening similar to the one I experienced so many years ago.

It was not just my study in India that informed the pages within. It was the years upon years of self-discovery combined with wisdom from masters, teachers, and loved ones across the globe. This book had many renditions as the world of 2020 continued to change, and my relationship to myself and my Kundalini practice ebbed and flowed along with the tides. With each layer of self discovered, we build upon the lessons of before. I would be remiss to diminish my training in Pilates, Kundalini, and plant-based nutrition, for they each informed the pages within. So did my years in corporate America, the loss of my mom to cancer, the ending of my marriage, miscarriages, experiences with sexual harassment, abuse, personal traumas, and every not-so-pretty idiosyncrasy that has made me who I am today. Each up and down has shaped my learning, whether via higher education or the school of life.

This Is a Judgment-Free Zone

The masses of the modern world may not have been open to the life-altering changes of Kundalini prior to the global pandemic, but now, more than ever, we need its energy. This journey you are embarking on is a judgment-free zone. Whatever occurred prior, all that will occur during, and anything that might occur after are all a beautiful part of the ride. There will be ups, downs, sideways steps, and zigzag movements. Sometimes we falter. Other times we soar. You are here because there is something within these pages for you—an insight, healing, knowledge, exercise, or dialogue that will serve your highest good.

How you show up to your practice will differ from day to day. Some days it will be meditative; others, emotionally exhausting. Regardless of what transpires, know that it is for your highest and best. There is not a Subagh Kriya performed where I do not have tears streaming down my face or a One-Minute Breath where I don't break into a yawn mid-practice. Through Kundalini, we move energy, and sometimes that energy is intense. Being perfect is boring, and pretending you are perfect is downright dangerous. So go ahead: yawn, cry, and scream at the top of your lungs. If you feel something bubbling up inside of you, let it out. Kundalini uses breath, movement, and a combination of different modalities to stir up what lies dormant within. Stirring things up so that they rise and can be released is, after all, the point of the whole thing.

Every range of emotion moves through the body. It is when you pretend that everything is okay by pushing down thoughts and feelings that you cause disease in the body. If this has been your pattern in the past, I will not pretend this experience will be a breeze for you. Kundalini will be intense. Most likely *really* intense. With regular practice, you will unlock those walls of protection that keep the unwanted emotions at bay. Those emotions will need a place to go, and my suggestion is to surrender. Feel the feelings. Surrender to the fact that every emotion, deemed good or bad, is part of the human experience. We cannot have light without dark or dusk without dawn. Take the "could have," "would have," and "should have" out of the experience. Stop blocking yourself from your greatness because you fear the unknown.

Whether or not you realize it, you came to this book for healing. The fact that you are here is an act of self-love. You loved yourself enough to invest in this journey; now, I encourage you to love yourself enough to remain open-hearted through the process. It may not always look pretty, but it will be the truth. I pray this serves you, your highest good, and the highest good of the world. Let's step into this safe space together. No judgment, just love.

How This Book Came to Be

New Year's resolutions can be powerful tools, often acting as a match that lights a fire underneath you. But what happens when this well-intended match has the opposite effect, burning the house down instead of being a shining catalyst for change? My story surrounding New Year's resolutions is the latter. For five consecutive years, I made the resolution to create a daily meditation practice, and for five straight years, I failed epically.

If you visited New York City in the early 2010s, there was a strong chance you were a stone's throw away from a conversation involving meditation at all times. Toted as the secret sauce to life, everyone who was anyone was talking about it, writing about it, and singing its praises. From Harlem to Brooklyn and everywhere in between, meditation was the drug of choice, and everybody wanted a hit. There was always someone raving about meditation's life-changing medicine or cursing its difficulty. It became apparent to me that there was something magical about this practice, yet despite my attempts, I could not harness this medicine in my daily life. With each passing year, the ability to quiet my mind eluded me.

A stressed-out New Yorker, I was working sixty-to-eighty-hour workweeks. I embodied zero work-life balance, resulting in a downward spiral of my mental and physical health. I began dropping weight from the sheer fact that I "didn't have time" to eat, and when I did eat, my stomach was a wreck. I've suffered from the side effects of auto-immune diseases throughout my life, and as my overworked and overstressed lifestyle accelerated, my healing journey began to regress. Old symptoms flared up, relationships outside of the office screeched to a halt, and my ability to effectively perform my job diminished. As I approached year five of failed meditation attempts, on a weekday like any other, an email broke the monotony of my frustration and changed my life.

The email was from the Rubin Museum, a museum I had not heard of before, inviting me to that evening's event on meditation. I had been praying for help, and this email felt like the answer to those prayers. Within a few short hours I was en route to 17th Street, still unsure of what I had gotten myself into. It was not until I found my seat and quickly perused the pamphlet that I learned the evening included a showing of the docuseries *On Meditation.* The viewing was to be followed by a discussion between two panelists: one the author of a metaphysical text and the other a virtually unknown (at least compared to her star status today) Gabrielle Bernstein.

As the auditorium filled and the presentation began, Gabby took center stage, informing us that she would "ground us" into the room. At her direction, hundreds of us raised our arms into the air in unison. She instructed us to stretch them into a high V, our thumbs actively plugged into the Universe. The direction seemed strange but, willing to try anything once, I complied. Together, all of us began intensely breathing in and out as our arms remained above our heads. The Kundalini technique lasted three minutes, concluding as we lowered our hands to our knees, sitting quietly for what was one of the most miraculous minutes of my life. As I opened my eyes, I turned to the person next to me and exclaimed, "I just meditated! What is this magic, and how do I get more of it?" Via the power of one three-minute Kundalini kriya, meditation no longer eluded me. I had finally, after years of searching, experienced its bliss.

Over the next four years, I sought out Kundalini classes throughout the city. My favorite was held in a studio just south of Gramercy Park. Every weekend I centered my Sunday around attending this class. Living in the West Village, my commute was, at best, forty minutes each way, turning this hour-long class into a three-hour excursion. The profound transformations I experienced were worth every second. It was in these classes that I felt something unexplainable. My heart lifted and my mind expanded. Emotions previously pushed down and buried came to the surface. Each session was physically challenging in ways I never could have anticipated.

Living and hustling in New York City had pushed me to my limit. Almost daily, I dreamed of leaving it all behind, darting off to India in the middle of the night. Kundalini was the only thing keeping my head above water, and the more aware I became of the emotions lying dormant within, the stronger the pull to pack my bags and immerse myself in its wisdom became. Because I was not fully tapped into my intuition at this juncture, I struggled to put into words how overwhelming—and at the same time, debilitating—this feeling was. I knew something needed to change and yet, for the life of me, I could not determine what that "thing" was.

Feeling more lost than ever, I shared the pendulum swing of my emotions with my Kundalini teacher. Her wisdom reframed the extreme swing of New York life I was living. She affirmed that yes, one solution could be to forsake the fast-paced city and retreat to a simpler, more isolated life. We could follow the guru path before us, living on mountain tops, meditating, and finding serenity in nature. We could isolate ourselves from the hustle and bustle of modern life, but how would that impact the greater good? What would it look like to take a different approach—to raise the vibration of the collective? What if we kept our corporate jobs, staying right where we were, but brought this medicine to those who might not otherwise have access to it?

I contemplated her words. If I left New York, what about the people I left behind? Those who were equally as stressed, overworked, and at the end of their ropes? How would selling my possessions and leaving my life in the rearview mirror bring others the peace and healing they also deserved? Could I learn to be of service right where I was? It would take many more years of internal work to cultivate the ability to be of service, but at that moment, I understood the truth: My soul is not one to retreat. I am not one to run away from a fight, especially if that fight is with myself.

A few years later, I found myself on that plane to India. I left the corporate world behind to study Kundalini's magic. What transformed my daydreams of years prior into the moment I chose to go to India was the intent. The adventure was no longer rooted in escapism; this trip came to fruition when I decided to dedicate my life to sharing the magic of Kundalini with the world. I needed to go back to the source, and not just for my education. My soul called me to India so that I could be of service to others. This book is the by-product of that soul's calling.

That fateful day in cold and gloomy New York City changed my life. It would be one of my greatest joys if this book could do the same for you. To me, books are living, breathing entities with spirits, each their own. Even if you never read past this paragraph, the heart, soul, and boundless amounts of love I put into this book's pages will vibrate outward from wherever it resides. Where intention goes, energy flows, and by purchasing this book and opening its pages, you have already started the process of absorbing its wisdom.

One
Kunda What?
(Kundalini Basics Explained)

WHAT IS YOGA IN the modern age? Stretchy pants? A room heated to over 100 degrees? Is it categorized as a workout, a spiritual practice, or all of the above? It's challenging to know what yoga is, let alone how or why to practice. With so many variations, where does one begin?

There are lineages, such as Bikram yoga, that perform a set sequence of postures. A quick search of "What makes Bikram yoga different?" provides a clear picture of what to expect when executing this type of yoga anywhere in the world: "Bikram yoga consists of the same twenty-six poses and two breathing exercises performed in the same order every class for exactly ninety minutes."[2] A clear, concise description. Ninety minutes of two types of breathing techniques and twenty-six postures.

Sounds easy enough, but what happens if you replace Bikram with Kundalini yoga in the search bar? One description of Kundalini yoga read: "Kundalini yoga was designed to awaken energy in the spine."[3] Straight away, the confusion begins. Awaken energy in the spine? What energy is held in the spine, and what does it mean to awaken it? The next sentence is only moderately less confounding: "Kundalini yoga classes include meditation,

---

2. Tripp, "Hot Yoga vs Bikram Yoga."

3. Beirne, "Yoga."

breathing techniques such as alternate nostril breathing, and chanting, as well as yoga postures."[4] That is a lot of information in one sentence, and not all of it clear.

The search engine response for Bikram yoga told us exactly what to expect. It included how long the class is, the number of breathing exercises, and number of postures. There is no need to search further. The response to a question about Kundalini did the opposite. It raises questions such as: Meditation? What type of meditation and for how long? Breathing techniques, such as alternate nostril breathing? What is alternate nostril breathing? Are there also twenty-six yoga postures in Kundalini? More? Fewer? The list of questions could go on and on. The problem isn't that this search is confusing, it is that this response is the norm. Yes, Kundalini is all of those things, but with such broad and vague descriptions, it is no wonder Kundalini remains the stuff of legend. Perhaps Kundalini yoga defies a simple definition.

Throughout this book, I demystify Kundalini by removing the confusion. The postures, meanings behind the words, length of exercises, and much more are explained. I also discuss the personal challenges that might surface while on your Kundalini journey. Kundalini is more than an activity to get you in shape. It works subtly to change your body from the inside out. Bench-pressing might lead to great pecs, but Kundalini results in great pecs, an open heart, and so much more. Before we dive too deep into the details, let's start at the beginning. What are the basics of Kundalini?

Who? What? When? Where? Why? And How?

We begin with the most fundamental questions. Who can practice Kundalini? What do you need to practice? When should Kundalini be practiced? Why do we practice? And how long is a Kundalini practice? Let us begin our Kundalini investigation.

Who Can Practice Kundalini?

Anyone! Kundalini is a yoga practice accessible to all. As long as you can move your arms, breathe without strain, and find a comfortable seat, you can perform Kundalini. If your mobility is limited, there are exercises where no arm movements occur, as well as modifications that provide adaptations for the ones that do. Flexibility is not a prerequisite, nor is the ability to bench-press your body weight. Some postures build physi-

---

4. Beirne, "Yoga."

cal strength, but building physical strength and showing up physically strong are two entirely different things.

The majority of Kundalini techniques occur in a seated position, instructed to be performed on a meditation pillow or mat. This is recommended based on the yogic science behind the work, but that does not mean it is the only way to proceed. If physical limitations are present—be it in your body or environment—the techniques can be performed in an alternate position, like a chair. Modifications are given at the end of most methods, making them accessible and achievable regardless of physical limitations.

What Do I Need to Practice Kundalini?

Just you! Some things can aid your practice, such as a meditation pillow, but the only requirement for most techniques is you. When performing any form of exercise, comfortable clothing is encouraged, as well as props such as a block or mat, but none are necessary to complete the activities. If a pillow is cued to elevate the hips, grab one from the couch or bed. Though I would love to travel consistently with my meditation pillow in tow, this is rarely the case. Most of the time when I'm not at home, my practice begins by sitting up straight in my bed or on the couch and utilizing whatever pillow is within arm's reach. As long as you are comfortable and can perform the techniques without physical pain, you are cleared to proceed.

When Should Kundalini Be Practiced?

Whenever! Any practice is better than none, and the techniques within are accessible at any time of the day. They are here to aid you whenever you might need them. I highly suggest picking a time of day that works with your schedule to commit to your practice. Not only will this cultivate consistency and discipline, but it will begin to train your nervous system to drop into a parasympathetic state. Also known as *rest and digest*, when the parasympathetic nervous system is activated, your heart rate slows and areas where you typically hold tension relax.[5] By committing to the same time each day, you build muscle memory within your body, cueing this parasympathetic response that allows you to drop into a meditative state more easily.

---

5. *Encyclopaedia Britannica Online*, s.v. "Parasympathetic nervous system," updated September 6, 2019, https://www.britannica.com/science/parasympathetic-nervous-system.

With this commitment to yourself, you train your body to relax every time you practice. The additional benefit is that when you choose to implement Kundalini techniques outside of this set daily time, your muscle memory automatically kicks in. With each daily practice, you are training your body to relax. Every time you practice Kundalini, your body is subconsciously cued to begin rest and digest.

Where Should Kundalini Be Practiced?

Anywhere! Another selling point for Kundalini is that it does not need to be done anywhere in particular. Some techniques do require a bit of room to move around, but most can be done at any time, in any place. I have performed Kundalini at work, in the car, in airplanes, in hotel rooms, on subways, and in nature. You may not have the space to raise your arms in an airplane, but you can perform a One-Minute Breath.

One of the benefits of the modern age is connecting digitally regardless of your physical location. Practicing within a community is a beautiful experience. If you do not have access to a Kundalini studio, you can still cultivate an online community. There are like-minded individuals ready to join you in this practice worldwide, should you have the courage to seek them out. As Rumi said, "What you seek is seeking you." Kundalini helps you cultivate the fortitude to act on those desires.

Why Should I Practice Kundalini?

To come home to yourself! Regardless of where you reside, connection with the outside world is accessible, now more than ever. Yet, if you were to look inward with a vulnerable honesty, where are some of these connections resulting in a disconnection from yourself? Each time you sit to practice, you call home the pieces of yourself scattered throughout the ether. With every interaction, you leave a small imprint of your essence behind—the anger toward the person who cut you off on the highway, or the human encroaching on your personal space while on the subway. It is these fragmented pieces of yourself that you call home with each practice.

What you do not own owns you, and unresolved emotions wreak havoc on the mind, body, and spirit. Kundalini stirs up the feelings lying dormant within. The subconscious houses old thought patterns and experiences. *Subconscious* means under consciousness. Below your awareness, there is an entirely different story, running on a continual loop, calling the shots. We make decisions from the narrative of the subconscious each day— the proverbial eight-year-old within, ruling even the smallest decisions played out in everyday life. Kundalini shakes you up from the inside out, bringing these emotions and experiences to the surface. With Kundalini, you move the subconscious to the conscious, unlocking what lies dormant within so that it may be healed.

How Long Is a Kundalini Practice?

It varies! Unlike Bikram yoga, Kundalini is not always precisely ninety minutes. Most of the Kundalini Kriyas are much shorter. The exercises within have been chosen not only for their ease and powerful results but also for their duration. There is not an exercise within this book that is longer than fifteen minutes. Most of them are one- or five-minute techniques. The results of these short experiences are what hooked me on Kundalini in the first place. My first experience with Kundalini, as mentioned in the introduction, lasted a mere three minutes. At the end of those three minutes, I sat in a one-minute meditation. Three minutes of Kundalini was all it took for me to meditate for the first time in my life. For less than five minutes of effort, I was able to quiet my mind and open my consciousness to an entirely new way of being. This is Kundalini's beauty—it is a pinpointed, intentional practice with maximum results in a minimum amount of time.

Common Kundalini Terms

As we dive into Kundalini's practice, let's discuss the fundamental terms you will hear, not only in this book but in any yoga lineage. The chapters within examine each in greater detail, but without a solid foundational knowledge, one could easily get lost in the newness of it all.

Kundalini presents as mystical with vocabulary that is in another language, particularly when words are thrown about as if you should already know their meaning. As we review some of the most common yogic terms, you will build a foundational understanding of the vocabulary found throughout this book, setting yourself up for success. You can find many more terms in the glossary at the back of the book.

Asana

An asana is a posture. If you have attended a yoga class, you have most likely heard postures cued in Sanskrit. Tadasana (Mountain Pose), Utkatasana (Chair Pose), Trikonasana (Triangle Pose), or Savasana (Corpse Pose)—the end of each word contains the word *asana*, signifying a body posture. It is common to hear someone speak of their "asana practice." Often used interchangeably with the word *yoga*, an asana practice is simply the practice of yoga's postures. Asana, in this context, is used as a generalization of one's yoga practice.

Bandha

Bandhas are yogic locks. These are specific constriction locations in the body where particular muscles are squeezed and engaged in a locked position. Bandhas are so integral to the Kundalini yoga practice that an entire chapter of this book is dedicated to them.

Not seen with the naked eye, these muscle contractions are different than the flexing of a bicep. Kundalini works on moving the energy and muscles found within—the deep muscles rarely highlighted in modern exercise practices of today. If you are not used to squeezing these muscles, the action of engaging the bandhas may seem difficult at first, but once you get the hang of it, the impact of your practice will skyrocket.

Chakra

Chakras refer to the seven energy centers that run vertically along the midline of the body. The first chakra starts at the spine's base, moving upward in numeric order to the head's crown. It is common for the colors associated with each of these centers to be shown in diagrams. The chakras follow the colors of the rainbow, beginning with the first chakra and the color red up to the seventh chakra, the color violet.

The chakra system is integral to Kundalini's practice as the Kundalini energy within each of us is located just below the spine's base, directly underneath the root chakra. The unblocking and awakening created during Kundalini's practice moves Kundalini energy upward through the chakra centers.

Drishti

The drishti is the location of your focused gaze. In a traditional vinyasa flow, finding your drishti is often cued during the standing posture series. By focusing your gaze on a single point, you aid in gaining and maintaining your balance. In a physically challenging yoga flow, this gaze is vital to ensure you remain upright instead of toppling over while in postures such as Tree Pose.

The location of one's drishti is given in virtually every Kundalini exercise. Most often cued is to focus one's gaze in and up toward the third eye, instructing you to close your eyes and gently roll them up and back until the gaze rests just above the eyebrow center. This spot, the ajna chakra location, is said to be the window to intuition.

Kriya

A kriya strings together a sequence of asanas, or postures, to create an intended effect. Performing a kriya means there will be more than one posture in the series. Kundalini uses yogic science to stir up and manifest an intentional outcome within the body, rippling its effect into your environment. As an example, Subagh Kriya brings forth wealth and prosperity. The kriyas within this book outline the result so that you may pick an exercise that most appropriately suits your current situation and needs.

Kundalini Awakening

A snake coiled three and a half times just under the spine's base is the visual representation of one's Kundalini energy. Said to be the source of our most extraordinary power, Kundalini energy is the location of your highest, most authentic self. A Kundalini awakening occurs when this energy ignites. This energy, as depicted by the snake, uncoils, crisscrossing the chakras as it rises up the spine. The chakra's power is activated as the Kundalini energy ascends. Once Kundalini energy reaches the last chakra, one is said to achieve samadhi, the ultimate state of bliss and enlightenment.

Mantra

A mantra is a word or group of words sung or chanted to invoke an intention. Kundalini mantras are almost always in Sanskrit; their meanings are more likely to be decoded into your language of origin by the instructor, not as a part of the Kundalini practice. Mantras are an invocation that uses the vibration of words to create a cause and effect. The most common Kundalini mantras start and end the practice, signaling the intent to begin and end. The vibrations created through the chanting of mantras are said to be more powerful when done in community. Therefore, it is common to see large rooms of individuals chanting the same mantras to evoke a desired collective effect.

Mudra

A mudra is a gesture. Most often, the mudras used in Kundalini are those utilizing the hands, but not every mudra is a hand mudra. A subtle energy, the use of mudras is said to change the environment slowly over time. Backed by yogic science, each variation changes the meaning of the gesture. The most common yoga mudra is Gyan Mudra, which brings the thumb's tip to the pointer finger's tip. This mudra is commonly used as a meditation mudra across all yoga lineages.

Nadi

Nadis are the more than 72,000 energy centers flowing throughout the body. Like thousands of thin branches from the base of a tree, these energy fibers send information throughout the body. This symbolic tree runs vertically along the spinal column, which houses the chakra system. Each of the nadis connects through at least one chakra, transmitting information from this central hub throughout the body's extremities. Out of the 72,000+ nadis, three main nadis are utilized in Kundalini: the ida, pingala, and sushumna. Just as the veins carry blood, the nadis carry the manifestation of prana.

Prana

Prana is the breath. The air that enters the body oxygenates the blood and removes toxic by-products from your system. Prana is referred to as life force energy for, without air in your lungs, you would cease to exist. Breathing, or the art of intentionally moving your breath, is a foundational component of a Kundalini practice. Unlike a vinyasa flow, where only one type of breathing is cued (Ujjayi Pranayama), Kundalini uses multiple breathing techniques throughout the practice. Learning different ways to breathe and how to breathe correctly is fundamental to the execution of Kundalini.

Pranayama

Pranayamas are breathing techniques used to move oxygen in and out of the body. Breathwork is done with the intent of awakening the Kundalini energy within you. Each method uses the manipulation of air to create a desired result. In Kundalini, breathing techniques are performed on their own, as well as during physical movement. Pranayama instruction informs the student what breathing exercise to utilize, either on its own or in tandem with a physical practice. Based on yogic science, the type of breathwork for a kriya always remains the same, specific to each exercise. Each instructor will cue the same breathing technique per kriya regardless of where, when, or with whom you practice.

Sacred Numbers

The sacred numbers one, three, five, seven, nine, eleven, twenty-one, twenty-seven, fifty-four, and 108 are found throughout Indian tradition. Thought to hold unique energy, these numbers repeat throughout yoga culture. For example, out of the 72,000+ nadis, three are noted as the most important. There are five pranayama divisions and seven chakras.

The importance of the sacred numbers is amplified in the science of Kundalini kriyas. The exercises in this book are in one-, three-, and eleven-minute increments, boosting these sacred numbers' power.

Sanskrit

Deriving from Vedic Sanskrit, Sanskrit is the ancient language in which all yogic philosophies originated. Documented as far back as 2000 BCE, it is one of the oldest languages on earth.[6] Still used in the modern world throughout all yogic sciences, aspiring yoga teachers cannot complete their certification without first demonstrating knowledge of their field of study in this ancient language. With each mantra, asana, mudra, pranayama, and kriya's original name in Sanskrit, it is common for yoga instructors to cue the technique first in Sanskrit, followed by the translation in the practitioner's native tongue.

How Kundalini Yoga Came to the West

The individual credited with bringing Kundalini yoga to the West is a man by the name of Yogi Bhajan. Born Harbhajan Singh Khalsa, Yogi Bhajan left his home country of India in 1968 for North America. Combining traditional Kundalini teachings with his Sikh heritage and tantric theories, Yogi Bhajan created a Kundalini lineage all his own. He took up residence in Los Angeles, where his style of Kundalini quickly gained popularity. In 1969 he founded the Healthy, Happy, Holy Organization, or 3HO. With over 300 centers in more than thirty-five countries, Yogi Bhajan's yoga brand has become widespread and prominent.[7] In today's modern world, if you have taken a Kundalini yoga class in any major city, it was most likely in the lineage of Yogi Bhajan.

Many of the experiences identified today as uniquely Kundalini are variations of the practice incorporating Yogi Bhajan's Sikh heritage. For example, it was not unheard of to

6. Chislett, "What Are the Oldest Languages on Earth?"

7. Sikhnet, "Yogi Bhajan."

wear turbans in one's Kundalini practice before Yogi Bhajan entered the scene in 1969, but he did make it customary. In Sikh tradition, both men and women wear turbans, an approach maintained by Yogi Bhajan and quickly adopted by those who practiced with him. The mantra "Ong Namo Guru Dev Namo" is derived from Yogi Bhajan's Sikh heritage and is commonly used to tune in or signify the beginning of one's Kundalini practice, just as "Sat Nam" is utilized as an ending invocation. We will discuss these mantras and their meanings in greater detail when we explore mantras in chapter 10.

Bhajan became famous, partly because he took this ancient lineage and distilled it in an easily digestible way. He explained techniques with verbiage the modern world could understand while breaking down the practice of Kundalini into shorter segments. As the Zen proverb states, "You should sit in meditation for twenty minutes every day—unless you're too busy; then you should sit for an hour."[8] Through his unique type of Kundalini, Bhajan found a way to squeeze an hour of meditation into twenty minutes, not the other way around. His yoga style incorporated the traditions of longer classes and devotions, introducing techniques that took three, five, and eleven minutes. Kundalini was no longer something one could only do if they dedicated their lives to the practice; it became something one could incorporate into their daily life.

The founding of 3HO occurred in 1969, the same year as Woodstock. This three-day peace and music festival is still considered one of the most significant cultural events of the twentieth century. Peace, love, and all things hippie were at the core of America's social climate change, and as Americans looked toward love over hate, the popularity of yoga began to rise. If you have any doubt that Bhajan's timing could not have been more ideal, the hit song "Aquarius/Let the Sunshine In (The Flesh Failures)" spent six weeks at number one on the US *Billboard* Hot 100.[9] This pop-culture phenomenon referencing the Age of Aquarius topped the charts at the exact moment Bhajan founded 3HO, and the US was swept away in the magic of making love, not war. Bhajan's Sikh heritage, where one's hair remains uncut and vegetarianism is a fundamental value, found itself in direct alignment with the time's energy. Yoga was on the rise worldwide, and Yogi Bhajan was virtually the only Kundalini yoga teacher in the West.

---

8. Daily Meditate, "Meditation Quote 3."

9. "Hot 100 Turns 60."

What's With All the White?

If you enter a Kundalini yoga class and find yourself surrounded by individuals dressed in all white, you have most likely entered a session in the tradition of Yogi Bhajan. Though wearing white during one's spiritual practice is nothing new, Bhajan is responsible for wearing head-to-toe white in Western Kundalini. Believing the color white expanded one's aura by at least one foot, Bhajan taught that this distance allowed for the filtration of negative influences, therefore protecting the wearer from unwanted energy. He also spoke of white as an exercise in awareness: because it is difficult to keep clean, white clothing challenges a person to stay mindful and present while wearing it.[10]

The use of white in spiritual practices spans religions throughout the globe. While studying in India, a few of my teachers wore white or lighter clothing from time to time, but rarely all at once. There is no enforcement that Kundalini yogis must wear white, although the teachers are encouraged to wear white. This is because Yogi Bhajan believed wearing white was thought to be a way of practicing consciousness. Outside of Yogi Bhajan's lineage of Kundalini, all white—including white head dressings—is not consistently worn. This is not to say that the emotional, spiritual, and psychological benefits of wearing all white should not be considered, however.

Cognitive psychology reinforces the wearing of white, noting that marketing and branding campaigns use white to symbolize purity, freshness, and cleanliness.[11] No different from the intention in many religious ceremonies, white is thought to be capable of wiping the slate clean, providing a pure vessel for spiritual work to occur. As Yogi Bhajan's popularity grew, white clothing adorned with a white turban became Kundalini's unofficial uniform. Because Yogi Bhajan was the Kundalini movement leader and the most famous Sikh in the West, this uniform crossed into Western Sikh custom. Today, most Western Sikhs (Kundalini practitioners or not) are often identified through their all-white attire. Yogi Bhajan was not the only individual to stress the benefits of wearing all white.

As you move forward in your Kundalini practice, please do not feel as if an all-white wardrobe is necessary to proceed. No uniform is required, as we are each whole and perfect just as we are. With that being said, should you feel tired or depressed, I suggest testing the power of color by wearing at least one white article of clothing. You will likely be surprised by how quickly your mood lifts and the energy within you changes. If the

---

10. Teachings of Yogi Bhajan, "Yogi Bhajan's Words on Wearing White."

11. Cherry, "Color Psychology of White."

thought of wearing white feels uncomfortable, begin by choosing a lighter color instead. Get creative and have a little fun. Evoking the energy of receptiveness still occurs with light colors, particularly when you feel comfortable in your skin. Bonus points if you tap into your uniqueness and call forth self-expression!

Exercises: Foundational Basics to Begin Your Kundalini Journey

The practices in this book are a combination of Yogi Bhajan's lineage and the foundational techniques of traditional Kundalini yoga. This book contains one-, three-, and eleven-minute kriyas. My goal with this book is to begin bridging the gap between the old and new worlds in both knowledge and process.

∽ Technique ∽
Sukhasana (Easy Pose)[12]

Duration: One minute.

Posture: The legs cross in toward the body with a straight spine as the palms rest on the knees.

Drishti: Eyes gently come to close while the internal gaze focuses on the third eye.

Technique: As the legs fold in toward the body and the spine straightens, the body's weight is balanced evenly across the sit bones. The head, neck, and spine are soft, just as are the lower extremities. There should be no pinching, pain, or discomfort in the body.

Action: Begin sitting on the ground, legs outstretched in front of the body, with a straight spine. Gently clasping one leg's shin, bring it in with the knee facing out. The calf and ankle come parallel to the body. Clasp the outstretched knee's shin and bring it in, placing the foot directly under the opposite knee. Adjust the foot of the first leg so that it is located under the opposite knee.

Modifications: If sitting upright with crossed legs feels uncomfortable, try utilizing a prop to elevate the hips. Pain in the hips will cause the spine and shoulders to round, making it impossible to sit with a straight spine. Using a yoga block will provide a firm foundation. A pillow or rolled-up yoga mat offers a softer experience. Try different

---

12. *Su* = Good. *Ka* = Space. *Asana* = Posture.

mediums at alternating heights to find a position that allows you to sit comfortably with a straight spine.

Variations: When open palms rest on the knees, the posture is grounding, creating a closed loop that circulates all energy inward. Turning the palms to face the ceiling opens the loop, creating an environment of receiving. Should you feel that your thoughts are scattered, face the palms downward. This action transmutes anxiety by directing it inward instead of outward. If you need guidance, turn the palms up, opening the body to receive direction from the divine.

Checking the Technique: Imagine a string running from the spine's base up through the body and out of the head's crown. Imagine someone is gently pulling that string upward, releasing the compression between the spinal vertebrae. The shoulders soften as the shoulder blades move down the backside of the body. The neck lengthens, and the distance between the shoulders and the ears increases. The neck and head move backward in space as the vertebrae realign to stack on top of one another.

Benefits: Can reduce stress and provide mental clarity.

ᔐ *Technique* ᔑ
Drishti at the Third Eye[13]

Duration: One minute.

Technique: Drishti is a focused gaze. When one's vision focuses on the third eye, this means that with closed eyelids, one's gaze turns up to the center point of the forehead, in between and slightly above the eyebrows.

Action: The eyes gently close as one's focus turns in and up toward the third eye.

Checking the Technique: The third eye is the location of the ajna chakra, the chakra of enlightenment. As you focus your gaze toward this point, envision the window to the Universe opening to the beyond. When your physical eyes are closed, this mystical eye opens, allowing what is within and beyond to move seamlessly between worlds.

Benefits: Can focus attention, quiet the mind, and provide a deeper meditative state.

---

13. *Drishti* = Gaze, viewpoint.

⌒ *Techniques* ⌒
Marjariasana-Bitilasana (Cat-Cow)

Duration: One minute.

Posture: The body comes to all fours with the knees located directly below the hips and the wrists directly below the shoulders. All four corners of the palms touch the floor; the weight is evenly distributed between each finger, finger pad, and palm.

Drishti: The neck aligns with the spine, the gaze settling in between the hands. As the technique begins, the eyes gently close, and the gaze refocuses in toward the third eye.

Technique: Begin with all four contact points, evenly distributing the weight between the knees and palms. The tops of the feet press firmly into the earth, toes untucked. The abdomen is engaged, bringing the spine and neck into alignment. The elbows have a gentle bend, allowing fluid movement in the sequence.

Technique for Bitilasana (Cow Pose): The posture occurs in one long inhale. The belly button drops toward the earth as the crown of the head reaches up. There is a lengthening of the front of the neck, chest, and abdomen as the body arches back. The influx of oxygen causes the spine to lengthen, creating expansion throughout the body.

Technique for Marjariasana (Cat Pose): The posture occurs in one long exhale. The navel pulls in toward the spine as the chin tucks into the body. The head's crown moves downward as air leaves the body and rounds in toward itself. The undulation ends on an empty stomach with the belly button pulled up and in, abdomen engaged.

Action I: Begin moving through the postures, inhaling as the head's crown reaches up and the belly drops. Exhale as the head tucks and the back of the body moves toward the sky.

Repetition I: Move fluidly through cat and cow for one minute, lubricating and increasing the spine's flexibility.

Action II: Slow the undulation to perform two long cat-cows. On a deep inhale, broaden the chest, lengthening the torso and filling the lungs slowly as the body extends. With a slow, deep exhale, pull the belly button deep into the spine, dropping the head's crown toward the ground, expelling all of the air from the body. Inhale to neutral, eyes gazing in between the fingertips. Exhale, taking the tailbone to the heels and stretching the fingertips to the front of the room. The palms press against one another, and the forehead gently rests against the ground in child's pose.

Repetition II: Move through the inhale of cow posture and exhale of cat posture. Inhale to a neutral spine and exhale to child's pose.

Modifications: If neck issues exist, maintain the neck's alignment with the spine while transitioning through the movements.

Checking the Technique: Both positions are performed while the hips remain directly over the knees and the hands align below the shoulders. It is common to sink the weight into either the hands or the knees. This is alleviated by bringing your attention to the weight distribution of all four connections to the ground. Feel the weight evenly distributed between the palms and the knees. If the knees or wrists hurt, this is a sign to focus more on the core. Take the weight out of the wrists and into the abdomen, bringing a lightness to the extremities.

Checking the Technique for Bitilasana (Cow Pose): As the body arches upward in cow pose, imagine a friend's hands gently cupping the shoulders, guiding them to roll backward, away from the ears and down the backside of the body. Envision the distance between the shoulders and the ears expanding as the body lengthens, stretching the spine upward while opening the chest.

Checking the Technique for Marjariasana (Cat Pose): As the spine rounds into cat posture, envision the broadening of the back. The shoulder blades pull laterally away from the spine, allowing air to escape through the body's back expansively. Envision a friend softly placing their fingertips on the inside of the hips, pulling them toward the ceiling as you exhale. Pinching sensations lift as the body lengthens away from the knees.

Benefits: Opening of the front and back of the body, warming the body, which can result in reduced inflammation and injury. Can benefit spinal health as oxygenation and cleansing of the blood occurs.

༄ *Technique* ༄
Adho Mukha Svanasana (Downward Dog)[14]

Duration: One minute.

Posture: Feet are firmly planted on the ground, hip distance apart. Hands are shoulder distance apart, flat on the ground with the fingers spread wide and pointing away from the body. Move the palms one hand length forward and raise the hips toward the ceiling, creating an inverted V with the body.

Drishti: The neck remains in line with the spine, eyes gazing in between the toes.

Technique: Take care to ensure the body's weight is evenly distributed between the palms and the feet. The heels press toward the ground, stretching the body's backside as hips raise toward the sky while the hands remain firmly planted on the ground.

Action I: To come into the posture, begin on all fours with the hands flat on the floor and fingers spread wide. Wrists rest directly under the shoulders, the knees under the hips. The toes tuck under, creating an arc under the shins while the knees and toes remain touching the floor.

Action II: The belly button pulls in toward the spine as the hips lift high, straightening both the legs and the arms into the shape of an inverted V. The palms remain flat as the heels move closer to the ground.

Modifications: Pedal out the legs, bending one knee and then the other to stretch and lengthen the lower extremities. Bring a soft bend into the knees, extending and pressing down toward the earth, closer with each repetition.

Checking the Technique: It is easy to shift the majority of the body weight into the wrists. As you hold the posture, pay close attention to how the weight is distributed through the palms. Is the majority of the weight directly under the wrists, or are the palms and fingers also flat on the ground with an even distribution of weight throughout? As the posture intensifies, strain might build in the neck with a natural tendency to gaze

---

14. Some Kundalini teachers refer to downward dog as *triangle pose*. Logically, this makes sense, because when the body makes an inverted V, from the side it looks like a triangle. The posture known as triangle pose in other yoga lineages, such as Vinyasa, is not used in Kundalini. Therefore, if a Kundalini instructor cues to move into triangle pose, they are requesting you move into downward dog.

between the hands instead of the toes. Take care to gently shake the head and neck from side to side, releasing tension and strain before coming back into the posture.

Benefits: Muscle lengthening, which removes toxins and redistributes blood throughout the body.

∽ *Technique* ∿
Chaturanga Dandasana (Four-Limbed Staff Pose)

Duration: One minute.

Posture: The body lowers from a plank. Halfway down, the elbows come into alignment with the ribs.

Drishti: The eyes look in between the fingertips, maintaining a straight line from the base of the spine to the head's crown.

Technique: The body moves from a downward dog into a plank position. The entire body lowers, pausing halfway before rolling over the toes to propel the body forward, arching the crown of the head and spine backward as the arms straighten.

Action I: The body moves into a downward dog.

Action II: The body rolls forward as the hips raise and the chin tucks into the body. The head and body straighten as the shoulders come into alignment over the palms, the weight evenly distributed between the toes and palms.

Action III: The weight of the body shifts forward slightly from the toes. The core and legs remain engaged as the body lowers halfway, stopping when the elbows align with the ribs.

Action IV: The body begins to roll over the toes, shifting the weight forward. The eye gaze rotates toward the front of the room and up to the ceiling, bringing the spine into a reverse C shape at the top. The tops of the feet touch the earth, knees and hips hovering as the arms straighten.

Action V: The body rolls back over the toes. Momentum is created from the core's movement, lifting the hips high and back into a downward dog.

Modifications: From downward dog, drop the knees to the floor, engaging the movement of plank posture from the knees instead of the toes.

Checking the Technique: There may be a tendency to dump most of the body's weight into the wrists. Alleviate this strain by distributing the weight evenly in both downward dog and plank, activating the legs and core. Keep the neck aligned with the spine by paying close attention to your drishti. The movement will become more fluid as your strength increases, creating a wavelike motion to the flow.

Benefits: Can lengthen and strengthen muscles.

ᴄ~ *Technique* ~ᴏ
Balasana (Child's Pose)

Duration: One minute.

Posture: Begin on all fours. The hips lower toward the heels. The big toes connect, knees splay wide, forehead touches the earth, and arms stretch forward in a straight line away from the body.

Drishti: The neck remains in line with the spine, forehead touching the floor as the eyes gaze in toward the third eye.

Technique: The body moves backward in space from all fours until the sit bones come to rest gently on the heels and the forehead rests gently on the ground.

Action I: Child's posture is most commonly transitioned into from all fours.

Action II: The hips shift backward into space, coming to land on the heels as the toes touch and the knees spread wide. The torso rests between the knees as the forehead rests on the floor. The arms stretch forward, palms flat on the ground with the elbows elevated, hovering in a straight line.

Modifications: The knees may come together to touch, with the torso resting on the upper thighs. The arms rest beside the body as the fingertips reach toward the toes. The palms turn toward the ceiling as the shoulders roll inward in this restorative posture.

Checking the Technique: This is a restorative posture, and therefore the entire body should be relaxed (minus the active arms). The full amount of your weight should rest heavily against the ground.

Benefits: Grounding. This relaxed state can bring rejuvenation to the body.

∽ *Technique* ∾
Breath of Fire

Cautions: Do not perform if pregnant or during the menstrual cycle. Avoid if pregnant or suffering from high blood pressure. Perform on an empty stomach.

Duration: One minute.

Posture: Sit comfortably in an easy pose, with a straight spine and palms resting gently on the knees.

Drishti: The eyes gently close as the focus turns in and up toward the third eye.

Technique: With lips sealed, forcefully inhale and exhale through the nose, bringing the belly button to the spine.

Action: Inhale through the nose with a straight spine, filling the body with air from the spine's base. On a full exhalation, empty the abdomen forcefully, pulling the belly button to the spine.

Repetition: Repeat forceful exhalation for one minute with three to four breaths per second. Upon completion, the breath slows, returning to natural breathing. With the inward gaze remaining fixed on the third eye, begin meditation.

Checking the Technique: Loosen the stomach muscles to allow the breath to move in and out forcefully. The belly will expand to a ball, filling the abdomen thoroughly, and then retract inward. The heat will begin to build as the duration of the technique lengthens.

Benefits: Can increase lung capacity. Detoxifies the body, reduces mucus, and may minimize cold symptoms.

Two

Manifest Like a Yogi
(Routines to Create Your Practice)

PEOPLE'S LIVES ARE CENTERED around the rise and fall of the sun. We wake each morning ready to tackle the day's to-dos and go to bed each evening to recharge from the day's events. All too often, the bliss of restfully waking with the dawn of a new day eludes most. For as long as I can remember, I have dreamed of becoming a morning person, harnessing the power of an in-sync circadian rhythm, propelling me forward throughout my day. In the ancient days of yore, people's bodies synced with the light of the seasons, naturally producing melatonin, ebbing and flowing with nature's cycles.[15] As humans continue to live an unnatural life in a natural world, the ability to tap into the fluidity of nature diminishes. A restless night's sleep followed by a groggy morning becomes the norm. The cycle is perpetually fueled by the unnatural stimuli consumed to get through the day.

Because it is no longer the body's natural inclination, the days when we push past our morning paralysis, we are amply rewarded. Committing to greet the sun is a hurdle I have consistently vowed to climb, for though my brain may be under a fog upon arousal, my body is always ready to greet the day. Beginning anew, mentally clear and spiritually connected, ripples into a level of health otherwise unattainable. The generations that came before us understood the wisdom of an early rise better than most. Well into his

---

15. Suni, "Melatonin and Sleep."

eighties, my grandfather still rises at 5:00 a.m., tinkering in his workshop and tilling the soil of his garden—all under the moon's glow. Through the discipline of recommitting to becoming a morning person, you create profound transformation in your life.

A Yoga Training Schedule

In 2019, after a fourteen-hour flight and a seven-hour car ride, I arrived in Rishikesh, India, under the night sky. Tired, jet-lagged, and in need of a reprieve, it took two full days of travel to reach my destination, the location of my yoga teacher training. Our host greeted me with a warm late-night meal, a tour of the facility, and itinerary for the month ahead. The morning's classes began bright and early at 6:00 a.m. with a packed schedule throughout the day. I was given a glimpse of the weeks ahead. With the other students already asleep and the majority of my travel completed under the night sky, I dragged myself to bed, embracing my new home for the next month.

Kundalini Teacher Training Schedule	
6:00–7:00 a.m.	Pranayama / Meditation
7:00–8:30 a.m.	Yoga asana practice
8:30–9:30 a.m.	Tea break and breakfast
10:00–11:00 a.m.	Mantra
11:00–12:00 p.m.	Kundalini practical
1:00–2:00 p.m.	Lunch
2:00–3:00 p.m.	Anatomy
3:00–4:00 p.m.	Kundalini meditation
4:00–5:00 p.m.	Yoga principles / Philosophy / Patanjali yoga sutra
5:30–7:00 p.m.	Kundalini asana class
7:00–7:30 p.m.	Rest time / Free time

Kundalini Teacher Training Schedule	
7:30–8:30 p.m.	Dinner time
8:30–10:00 p.m.	Self-study
10:00 p.m.	Lights out

Each day in Rishikesh I woke at 5:30 a.m., rising with both the monkeys and the sun. By 6:00 a.m. my classmates and I gathered in the main yoga room with our mats, notebooks, and a willingness to learn. Our teachers warned the first week would be agitating as we adjusted to a new climate, time zone, and culture. The pressures of the rigorous schedule would cause us to want to throw in the towel by week two, followed by settling into a routine at week three. They also predicted that one month in, firmly rooted in our schedule, we would be overcome with the opposite inclination—our desire to do anything but leave.

I rolled my eyes at their warnings only to watch them unfold as predicted. As time progressed, I grew accustomed to the schedule, noticing as my body began to follow suit. I became hungry at the designated mealtimes and started waking without an alarm. I witnessed the emotional shift in my classmates as we ebbed and flowed through the process. Exhaustion during week one, anger at week two, the beginnings of a routine by week three, and, lastly, a sadness to leave as week four concluded. We did eventually acclimate to the changes around us, physically, emotionally, and spiritually. At the time, I did not connect the dots between why and how this experience was structured; the ancient knowledge of the yogis was imparted on us during our studies, but it was not fully ingrained into my psyche until a full change of the seasons later.

Yogic Science and Mother Nature

Pointedly crafted, my Kundalini teacher training took one month to complete. The weeks were structured to build upon one another, much like this book, first providing baseline knowledge to create a solid foundation. The program factored in intellectual progression while considering the emotional evolution that would occur as we proceeded. There is a reason we were warned of the emotional rollercoaster soon to occur upon arrival—just as the tides ebb and flow with the moon's cycle, so too would our emotions as we progressed on this profoundly spiritual path.

The science of yoga works hand in hand with astrology, utilizing the power of the planets to create change and invoke enlightenment. When we discuss mudras in chapter 8, I will introduce the connection between each finger and its corresponding planet. As this connection is explored, how we utilize a planet's energy as a catalyst for change takes light. Not a planet but a natural satellite, the moon is a paramount force of the cosmos whose energy has an effect on both our bodies and planet earth. Moon phases can help us begin to explore our connection to the cycles of the planets as well as the seasons of Mother Nature. This is not a book about astrologic effects, but to begin, we explore the amplification of Kundalini's energy through the power of lunar phases.

New Moon

A new moon marks the beginning of a lunar phase. It is an astrological event that occurs when the sun, moon, and earth are in direct alignment. The energy of this alignment is harnessed in many traditions, such as a new moon circle: events in which individuals (be it by themselves or in a community) gather to release the weight of the previous month, setting forth intentions for the month ahead. The alignment of the sun, moon, and earth used to realign people's lives. Much like the twenty-eight-day structure of my yoga teacher training, day one of the lunar phase marks a moment of new beginnings when anything is possible.

This energy can be utilized at the beginning of any new endeavor. If there is something on your to-do list that always seems to remain on the back burner—say, creating a consistent spiritual practice—bring it to the forefront during the new moon. Set an intention to begin and maintain this action throughout the entirety of the lunar phase. You will notice that tasks that otherwise seemed arduous feel a bit lighter. With the extra pep in your step, beginning your Kundalini practice will feel fresh and new. Lean into this time of excitement and possibility, stepping forward on your Kundalini journey, burdens left in the past, fully present and open to the magic before you.

Full Moon

As you enter the middle of the month, so too follows the full moon. At the lunar phase's halfway point, a full moon occurs when the sun and moon are in opposition. The sun lights the moon fully due to its placement in the sky, shining a light on where things are out of balance in your life. Given a negative connotation in the folklore of yore, images of mythical creatures howling at the moon give way to feelings of fear and danger. At this juncture of the lunar phase, people wear their hearts on their sleeves. Caught in between the past and the present, a full moon is a time of reevaluation. Where have you gotten out of balance, and what lessons are you called to learn?

Contrary to some widely spread beliefs, this halfway point does not embody the energy of doom and gloom. Let's reframe these superstitions and instead witness a full moon as a time to celebrate how far you have come. Harness this energy by releasing the things that no longer serve you and recommitting to your goals. At this moment in your Kundalini journey, you might find that the commitment to your daily practice begins to wane. Now, with the knowledge that this has nothing to do with your resolve and every-thing to do with the course of nature, begin to breathe a sigh of relief. Shift your perspec-tive to view the full moon as a time to reflect on your journey with gratitude, combined with the empowerment to pivot your trajectory in a way that is more aligned with the person you are becoming. Life operates in duality. A full moon is the perfect opportunity to view both the past and the present from a place of neutrality.

Moon Cycles and Forming Habits

Anywhere from eighteen to twenty-eight days is often publicized as the duration of time needed to form a new habit. With the knowledge of a lunar phase (a full twenty-eight days) now under our belt, we can see that this widely spread ideal has something in com-mon with the lunar phases.

THE MAGIC OF A MONTH

We move through life in sync with Mother Nature's cycles. Each month the calendar cues us to a new chapter, the duration of a month varying between twenty-eight and thirty-one days. The average number of days in a month rounds out to between twenty-eight and twenty-nine days. The number of days in a lunar phase is virtually in sync with the number of days in a month. It is here we begin to understand the correlation between the two, our modern calendar's rhythm paralleling the phases of the moon.

Completing a task for a full twenty-eight days, the duration of a lunar phase, in order to solidify a new habit is sound reasoning, yet without intensive commitment—like the all-day-every-day rigidity of my Kundalini teacher training—it is unlikely that a person will create a new habit after only a month. During my time in India, I had one task: learning the wisdom of Kundalini. I was able to solidify this knowledge in my subconscious due to the intensity of this endeavor, yet should my mind have been elsewhere (like the ins and outs of everyday life), the same outcome would not have been achieved.

If you think back to the ghosts of New Year's resolutions past, you were most likely in the groove at the end of January, starting to see results from your daily discipline but nowhere near the end goal you sought to achieve. After one month of committing to a new habit, you've already overcome the first hurdle: that mid-month snag, the proverbial full moon, where what is new becomes hard just before the pressure releases. When you get to the end of an entire month, you begin to move forward with grit. This is not the time to let the foot off of the gas. Harness that momentum by charging ahead to day forty—the moment lasting change begins.

THE FORTY-DAY MOUNTAINTOP

If you have attended a Kundalini yoga class, you have likely heard a teacher's request to repeat a kriya for the next forty days. This is the intention to create lasting change through the daily discipline of executing the same exercise day in and day out. The results compound upon themselves, much like a wave, which builds as it flows. I like to think of this forty-day mark as the top of a mountain—the summit of a long, arduous, often rocky climb before the gentler experience of a descent. Not unlike the lunar phase mentioned previously, as a new month enters, the difficulty of a climb begins anew. This is also the moment when resolutions historically begin to fade. The resolve a person gained crossing the finish line of the first month wanes as they enter month two.

The lunar phase following a new moon is a waxing crescent. As the transit moves from alignment to opposition, the sun's light begins to illuminate the moon. Visually represented as a crescent shape in the night sky, we can quite literally see the pressure building. The energy of this cycle and the hurdles encountered during this phase build as the next full moon draws near.

With the knowledge of a lunar phase solidified, you are armed with the tools to conquer the forty-day mark mentioned by your Kundalini yoga teacher. As you break down that forty days as just another full moon, the path of what to expect is illuminated. Deflate some of the self-limiting beliefs you may have surrounding your ability to succeed by shifting your mindset to think of this as the second full moon of your journey rather than a full forty days of work. By connecting to nature and focusing your gaze, the task becomes less of an uphill battle, thought of as merely the next phase of the journey instead of as a mountain to climb.

The halfway point of a season, day forty, is when we begin to see life-altering results. Your goals, still very much at the forefront of your mind, start to become second nature. Yogic science teaches us that it takes a full forty days to establish the cadence of one's habit. Up until this point, you have diligently put in the work. Daily discipline shifts into a routine, creating your new normal. Represented by the top of a mountain, with an arduous climb behind you, day forty-one begins.

THE DESCENT

Officially over the mountaintop, at day forty-one, you begin the descent—your efforts now showing outwardly, physically, mentally, and emotionally. You slightly release the grip held around your goals. What was in your conscious mind begins to become unconscious. Just as this time in a lunar phase ushers in the waning crescent, so too does your resolve begin to wane. Revisiting the comparison to a New Year's resolution, think back to a goal you had and what its status was by Valentine's Day. Around this time of the year, during the second lunar full moon, did your resolve begin to fade? The descent, the days after day forty, separate life-altering change from the backslides of previous efforts. Your yogic tools are crucial as this shift begins to take root in your subconscious.

As a new pattern becomes more ingrained and effortless, we naturally relax and inadvertently allow the old way of doing things to seep back in. Unlike the times before, this time, allow your knowledge of yogic science to take center stage. Yogis understand that all things flow by following nature. Things may have gotten more difficult around the forty-day mark, but just as you began to feel relief after last month's full moon, so too will you begin to feel relief in the weeks that follow. Your journey toward a new way of doing things is a tidal wave, moving your emotions through your body with the power of the moon. Harnessing this energy, begin to flow through the process. With this new resolve, you recommit to your effort, knowing that the permanent life-altering results are in your sight. Begin to think about the future, intellectualizing that it takes nature a full ninety days to perform a permanent death and rebirth. Each season ushers in a new paradigm, like clockwork, four times a year.

DAY NINETY

Now tapped into the energy of a full lunar phase, our gaze broadens. Zooming out, connect the dots between the death and rebirth experienced in a month with the new life created in the span of ninety days. Honing in on this wave of change, curiosity begins to surround the seasons. Think about the transitions progressing through winter, spring, summer, and fall. How is it that Mother Earth continually reinvents herself, and is it possible for us to do the same? What roadblocks have you encountered that hold you back from this continual rebirth? Begin to wrap your mind around previous attempts. In the past, where have you failed? When did you succeed? Have there been junctures where you could taste victory, only to stumble just before the finish line? What is it about the successes that differ from the moments of *almost*? What is the key to reaching success on day ninety?

Instead of backsliding, rely on your yogic training to move forward to the finish line. Aware of the shift to the subconscious, begin to give yourself grace surrounding the times when you previously fell short. Get curious and begin to track your patterns. Did you stumble at day forty, the top of the mountain? Did you feel amazing around the midway point of a season, only to let your old subconscious programming take the driver's seat as your resolve relaxed in the weeks ahead? Remember, subconscious programming has been with you all your life. The majority of your decisions are made from old thought patterns and neural pathways. The attempt to create a new habit requires new neural pathways—quite literally, new synaptic connections within the brain—pathways that must be strengthened and reinforced. It won't happen overnight. Armed with the knowledge that even after two months of effort, it is the body's natural inclination to revert back to the old, safe, familiar way, offer yourself grace for when you have failed, combined with the strengthened resolve to push forward toward everlasting change.

With yogic tools at your fingertips, there is a realization that you are, in fact, divinely supported in your efforts toward change. Through yoga's awareness and mental fortitude, you consciously progress toward your goal. With Mother Nature as the guiding light and yoga as your spiritual running buddy, you can finally allow a habit to take permanent hold within your subconscious by day ninety. This is the time when your circadian rhythm and the other functions of your body naturally perform tasks. Through consistent effort, you have strengthened new neural pathways, quite literally rewiring your brain. You will no longer have to put so much effort into achieving your goal, this habit now the new normal. Your body's natural instincts will work for your highest and best good with this new habit solidified.

The Magic of a Season and Kundalini

As you awaken to these synchronicities you unlock the wisdom of your intuition, lying dormant within. Armed with the knowledge that it takes a full lunar phase to create the repetition of a new pattern, forty days for that pattern to become second nature, and ninety days to make a permanent change in your life, a light bulb turns on in the brain. Understanding these facts, you can begin to see your Kundalini practice as an aid to help you along the way.

With each new goal or resolution, you have an opportunity to amplify the effects and guarantee lasting results by selecting a Kundalini kriya to accompany the endeavor. If you want to break an addictive pattern, add in the Meditation to Heal Addictions each day to aid you along your journey. Are you looking for resilience? Commit to the Excel, Excel, Fearless Meditation for the next ninety days. Starting a new kriya in conjunction with any new goal amplifies the energy of both intentions. Harnessing the power of a season combined with the compounding energy of your Kundalini practice will result in a transformation far more significant than you could have ever imagined.

Wake Like a Yogi

Now that you understand the synchronicities between the body and the seasons, let's go deeper into our practice. We begin by diving into nuances to further hone the path toward success. Chronicle each day's events, beginning with your morning routine. Whether you are a morning person or not, we all start our day with one decision: when to rise. A gamut of choices immediately follows, and a windfall of brain-scrambling information comes at us before we even open our eyes. It's no wonder we have gotten tripped up in the past. Without a clear plan of action, how could we expect to succeed? You can sigh a breath of relief as you sync yogic and natural methodologies instead of succumbing to the overwhelm.

Looking back at the schedule outlined for my Kundalini training, each day began at 5:30 a.m. The thought of hearing an alarm go off this early might cause you to begin to yawn inadvertently, but for many a yogi, waking at 5:30 a.m. is considered sleeping in. While in India, the term *auspicious* was spoken regularly by our teachers. It most often referenced the ambrosial hours, the most auspicious time to practice. In Sanskrit, it is spoken as *brahmamuhurta*, or "the divine time." [16] Both Ayurvedic and yogic sciences

---

16. Satyananda Saraswati, *Kundalini Tantra*, 199.

believe that it is the two hours before the sun rises, between 4:00 a.m. and 6:00 a.m., that we come closest to God. The exact times vary as the seasons change, but the energy behind this theory remains. This is the time that we are able to tap into the knowledge of the Universe with supreme awareness. The two hours before sunrise are said to enable us to connect to the energy of creation. We are beginning anew, just as the day does, with the rising of the sun. This is an example of yoga yet again taking its cues from Mother Nature and life's natural order.

Amrit Vela [17]

During this auspicious time, the yogic collective most often execute *sadhana*, a daily spiritual practice.[18] Typically performed during the ambrosial hours, sadhana refers to any practice done consistently in pursuit of spirituality. Many temples and Kundalini studios open their doors freely to the public between 4:00 a.m. and 6:00 a.m., ensuring all in search of a deeper connection to the divine are welcome.

The benefits of performing a daily sadhana extend beyond the personal. These repetitive acts are believed to elevate the higher consciousness of all. Whether alone or in a group, as people cultivate connections to a higher power at the same time, an energetic ripple effect is created throughout the world. In Islam, Muslims carry out salat, praying five times each day. Halakah, or Jewish religious law, calls for Shabbat's weekly observance—just as Christian lineages maintain the tradition of attending church each Sunday. Regardless of the foundational beliefs, the profound energetic shift of these collective practices has been documented and performed throughout the ages. Their importance, backed by yogic science, is referred to as sadhana.

As you embrace your practice during the same hours each day, you begin cultivating a vortex of spirituality. Just as your body and circadian rhythm sync up as you repeat functions day after day, so too does your trust muscle's connection to the divine. The concept of building a trust muscle is similar to building the strength of any other muscle in your body. It is through continued, dedicated, and pinpointed effort that you gain physical strength. It is through repetition and intention that your trust in yourself, the divine, the Universe, and whoever and whatever you believe in increases.

---

17. *Amrit* = Ambrosia. *Vela* = Hours.

18. Satyananda Saraswati, *Kundalini Tantra*, 199.

After years of dabbling in meditation, it was not until I embarked on my first stay at an ashram that I experienced the magnitude of collective energy. The ashram was a location where, for over sixty years, individuals have flocked in the pursuit of spiritual seclusion. I was struck by the palpable collective force the site emanated. The ability to effortlessly drop into a meditative state having eluded me in the past, each time I prepared for a "sit," I found myself immediately in an altered state. As I spoke with an ashram leader regarding this phenomenon, he graciously reaffirmed my intuitive hunch. Many who had attempted meditation and failed previously found the ability to "drop in" to be instantaneous while on the grounds. The location was electric due to the devotional intentions of its visitors for over half a decade.

There was, in fact, something in the air. As I walked down the paths and placed my bare feet in the sand, it was as if I could feel the electricity of Mother Earth emanating through me. The ashram felt shrouded under a dome of white light—like a higher power directly connected to the land—offering a safe space for all who entered. The collective consciousness was tangible in this location like no other I have experienced. For the first time, I understood the magic of this routine: repetitive actions that take place at the same time each day in the same location. Upon arriving home, my first task was to create such a place in my space: an altar and a corner to meditate daily. As my practice grew, I began to feel the cumulative results of this routine, creating my dome of spirituality, continually reinforced with each daily practice.

The Purpose of the Yoga Mat

As you cultivate the location where you will perform your daily ritual or sadhana, you might begin to inquire why the yoga mat is essential. When sitting in meditation, a yoga mat, pillow, or block may not seem like a necessary component, yet there is a spiritual reason for its use. The Vedas, the most sacred yogic texts, teach us about the Lokahs, or fourteen universes. Of the fourteen universes, the lower seven correlate to what is below the earth. The middle three universes connect to Earth, and the top four connect above the earthly plane. The yoga mat, pillow, or block that separates you from the ground is intentionally used to protect your energy from moving down toward the lower universes.

People spend the majority of their time standing, walking, or sitting. In each of these activities, energy is pulled down toward the spine's base and the earth due to gravitational pull. As you become more aware of the power of your daily activities, you will begin to notice that even as you sit, you feel the world's weight on your shoulders. Energy is pulling down toward the base of your spine and, consequently, is placed on your sacrum. Wearing shoes can protect our energy from transferring to the earth beneath us, just as the act of walking barefoot in nature is considered grounding, connecting us directly to the energy of the earth. When we sit—whether in meditation, at a desk, or on a couch—we have something in between the body and the ground, protecting that transfer of energy, cultivating and recirculating life force back into us.

Your yoga mat is not only a tool for creating space for your asana practice but an integral part of setting the intention of your actions. You purposefully draw your prana, or life force energy, back into yourself, separated from the ground by your mat and cushion. As you recirculate these vibrations, you come home to yourself. Your mat or pillow helps you drop into this meditative state of transformation. It's a visual cue, signaling to your mirror neurons that it is time to begin. The energy of your mat is palpable as you engage. Each intention is transferring to what is beneath you, leaving a permanent vibration in the object and creating a more in-depth experience with each "sit."

Exercises: Manifest Like a Yogi

The following exercises aid in your ability to manifest like a yogi. These foundational concepts work toward putting the lessons of this chapter into practice, creating an intention to manifest positive transformation in your life and the lives of others. This chapter teaches the connection between the actions of one to the actions of all, harnessing the energy of the moon and Mother Nature. As you complete the following techniques, embrace the empowerment that comes from knowing that each effort to better yourself is also an act of betterment for all.

ᥬ *Technique* ᥬ
Ambrosial Hours

Duration: Eleven minutes.

Take the time to fill out each journal prompt fully before moving on to the next. Each section will take you approximately eleven minutes to complete. If the task seems too arduous to work through in one sitting, you can journal at different times throughout the day or separate the prompts by day. Give yourself grace surrounding any feelings of anxiety or overwhelm that might surface. Take the time you need to work through your ideal evening and morning routine in a way that feels authentic and empowering.

Journal Prompt I: What time do you turn out the lights?

Is your sleep consistent?

Do you fall asleep at the same time each evening, or is your sleep pattern varied?

Do you have an evening routine? If so, what is it? Document each step and the time it takes to complete each.

Journal Prompt II: Regardless of whether or not you currently have an evening routine, what would your ideal evening routine be? Write out each step in consecutive order, including how long each step would take. How long is the entirety of this routine, from the moment you begin to the moment your head hits the pillow?

Journal Prompt III: What did you discover about your evening routine? Is it dialed in, or are there areas where you are wasting time? Do you consider loading the dishwasher and preparing meals for the following day part of your evening routine? Are you happy with how you prepare for bed and with the quality of your sleep? Is there something about your evening routine that you would like to change?

Journal Prompt IV: Rewrite your ideal evening routine, remembering to include all items, not just those that begin in the bathroom or bedroom. Add in any evening routine items like straightening the couch cushions or taking the dog for a walk.

Journal Prompt V: Compare your current routine to your ideal routine. How far apart are the two? Is there anything else you would change about your ideal routine, or are you happy with the path forward? Is this new evening routine manageable? Or were too many tasks added to the queue, making it impossible to maintain? Are you making life more difficult, or are you setting yourself up for success? Are these items written down because you feel you *should* be doing them or because you actually *want* to do them?

Journal Prompt VI: Revise, streamlining the process. Bullet point each task and include time frames for their completion. What time would you need to begin your evening routine in order to get a full night's sleep and awake at your ideal arousal time?

The Next Twenty-Eight Days: For the next twenty-eight days, or a full lunar phase, commit to completing this evening routine. Commit to your routine from start to finish, beginning with the ideal time to wind down and then following your tasks in the order they occur. As you approach the twenty-eighth day, you will be confidently aware of the energy of the lunar phase aiding in your endeavor, with bonus energetic support awaiting you if you began this task on the first day of a new moon. Here you will view, in real time, the benefits of setting yourself up for success through your knowledge of yogic science. By syncing your routine with nature, you will begin to witness the life-altering ripple effect of change spilling into other areas of your life.

We address an evening routine first because without nourishing your body with proper rest, any task completed in the morning will seem futile and impossible to maintain. The exercises throughout this book will benefit from your dedication to setting yourself up for success. Rising before the sun is an admirable goal, but if your nighttime routine is varied and out of whack, so too shall be your morning. Dialing in your evening allows you to clarify what you need to do and when in order to set yourself up for success each day.

↶ *Technique* ↷
One-Minute Breath

Duration: One minute.

Posture: Sit comfortably with a straight spine. The chest lifts, heart protruding outward, and the shoulders gently roll back as the chin tucks slightly in.

Drishti: Eyes gently close with the internal gaze focused on the third eye.

Technique: Inhale the breath for a count of twenty seconds. Hold the breath for a count of twenty seconds. Exhale the breath for a count of twenty seconds.

Mantra: Instead of counting from zero to twenty, elevate your practice by mentally reciting "Sa, Ta, Na, Ma" with each count. "Sa" with count one, "Ta" with count two, "Na" with count three, and "Ma" with count four. Repeat "Sa, Ta, Na, Ma" five times, bringing the final count to twenty.

Action I: Inhale for a count of twenty, mentally reciting the mantra "Sa, Ta, Na, Ma" five times.

Action II: Hold the breath for a count of twenty, mentally reciting the mantra "Sa, Ta, Na, Ma" five times.

Action III: Exhale for a count of twenty, mentally reciting the mantra "Sa, Ta, Na, Ma" five times.

Repetition: Complete Actions I, II, and III, bringing the total practice time to one minute. Sit in a comfortable seated position with eyes closed and meditate upon completion.

Checking the Technique: As you recite the mantra "Sa, Ta, Na, Ma," you will notice that each syllable begins to sync with your heartbeat. Begin to pay attention to the parts of the breath performed with greater ease. Do you have less difficulty with the long, slow inhale? Is the holding of the breath problematic? Does the long slow exhalation leave you gasping for breath?

As you tune in to this one-minute exercise's ease or difficulty, begin to find similarities to the comfort and resistance mirrored in your everyday life. How can you continue to do this exercise throughout your day to bring balance and ease back into your life?

Benefits: Can reduce anxiety and lower the heart rate.

❧ *Technique* ☙
Swan Kriya

Cautions: Avoid if pregnant.

Duration: Three minutes.

Posture: Begin kneeling on the ground with sit bones pressing against the heels and the inner thighs engaged, touching one another.

Technique: The four postures are performed in a wavelike motion. The upper body moves through the sequence fluidly, while the legs remain stationary and engaged, pulling in toward the centerline of the body.

Action I—Posture One: As you kneel on the calves, your palms come to the ground, resting flat on either side of the knees. The fingers are engaged with weight evenly distributed throughout all four corners of the hands.

Action I—Posture Two: Begin to lower the crown of the head, diving forward and pulling the navel to the spine, creating a C-shaped curve with the body similar to cat pose.

Action I—Posture Three: As you move closer to the ground, the head's crown stretches forward until the navel touches the upper thighs. The forehead hovers just above the ground with the spine straight.

Action I—Posture Four: Begin to turn your head upward, the crown of the head reaching toward your heels. The neck lengthens and the spine starts to arch, creating an inverted C-shaped curve on your body's backside.

Repetition I: The arced spine of posture four flows seamlessly to the rounded spine of posture two. The movement repeats for three minutes.

Action II: Come to sit upright with your palms facing up, fingers intertwined and tips of the thumbs touching. The backs of your hands rest gently on your upper thighs. Take three deep breaths with your eyes closed, keeping your internal gaze turned in toward the third eye.

Repetition II: Three deep breaths followed by meditation.

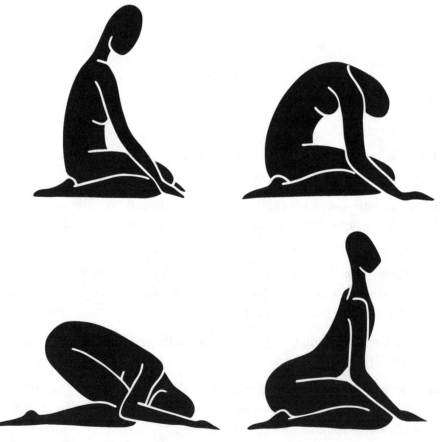

Swan Kriya

Modifications: The postures can be performed in a chair if kneeling causes discomfort or pain. The speed of the undulating motion may increase as you become more comfortable with the movement.

Checking the Technique: Envision performing these motions with the grace and fluidity of a swan dipping its beak in and out of the water. The spine's undulation will feel like a wave. The second posture of the sequence is similar to the movement of cat pose, with tailbone tucked and navel pressing deep into the spine, while the fourth posture is a similar motion to cow or cobra. The head moves backward and the back arches, heart opening through the front of the chest.

Benefits: Can aid in the clearing of negative emotions from the heart while providing clarity of the mind.

∽ *Technique* ∾
Sat Kriya

Cautions: Do not perform if pregnant or during the menstrual cycle.

Duration: Three minutes.

Posture: Begin kneeling on the ground with sit bones pressing against the heels and the inner thighs engaged. Often referred to as rock pose, the knees press firmly against one another.

Mudra: Hands are clasped and index fingers are outstretched, pressing against one another. Those who were born with male reproductive organs should cross the right thumb over the left. Those who were born with female reproductive organs should cross the left thumb over the right. The heels of the hands are pressed together. The arms straighten, reaching up over the head with pointer fingers pushing toward the heavens.

Drishti: The eyes close as the gaze turns toward the third eye.

Technique: The posture and mudra remain stationary throughout the kriya, creating an internal rhythmic wave as the mantra is spoken from the belly's pit.

Action I: Arms reach up, pointer fingers stretched toward the ceiling. Repeat the mantra "Sat Nam," chanting eight repetitions per ten seconds.

Repetition I: Complete the repetition of "Sat Nam" for two minutes. The arms remain straight, fingertips engaged the entire time, without dropping or relaxing the posture.

Action II: The eyes remain closed. Deeply inhale. With the mudra still intact, arms stretch up, squeezing the body's muscles tightly. Hold the breath, envisioning energy shooting out of the fingertips into the heavens. Exhale fully. On the exhale, hold the breath, applying the root lock by pulling the anus toward the navel.

Repetition II: Repeat the breathwork three times, bringing the total exercise time to three minutes. On the final exhale, release the arms in a sweeping arc-like motion, envisioning the cultivated energy bathing your auric field as the hands float to the earth at your side.

Checking the Technique: Focus your gaze on the crossing of the thumbs. Have you crossed the left thumb over the right, or do you need to adjust for the proper mudra placement? The pointer fingers press firmly against one another, arms straight and engaged, creating one long line of energy from the spine's base to the fingertips. Envision the tips of the fingers as an extension of the energy of your spine.

Benefits: Can tone the nervous system while improving the function of the internal organs through rhythmic massage.

Three
Shine Like a Yogi
(Chakras Demystified)

THE CHAKRA SYSTEM IS a cornerstone of most yoga lineages. Kundalini yoga uses the activation of the chakras to clear the path for your Kundalini energy to rise. By activating and balancing the energy centers of the chakras, we can utilize their wisdom to navigate our daily lives. When each chakra activates, so too do the nadis that reside within them, sending information through this nerve-like web throughout the body. As you practice Kundalini, you realign and perform techniques to awaken each of the chakras. Kundalini uses breathwork, movement, mantras, mudras, and intention to direct and circulate energy in these areas with the goal of a Kundalini awakening.

What Is a Chakra?

Chakra translates to wheel or circle. They are the medallions found on many a yoga poster, often denoted by each chakra's color and symbol. Not always depicted fully in the posters of today, each chakra contains six aspects. The first three—color, petals of the lotus, and geometric shape—are visible to the naked eye.[19] These are the images most people are familiar with, even if they do not quite know what they are viewing. Though you may have seen the chakras depicted thousands of times, with this knowledge you will now notice the color, number of petals, and geometric shapes within each diagram.

---

19. Satyananda Saraswati, *Kundalini Tantra*, 116.

Chakra aspect number four, the *beej*, or seed mantra, uses the power of sound to amplify the energy of each chakra. These two-letter mantras correlate with a note on the musical scale, utilizing a specific tone and vibration to amplify this sound. Singing bowls can also activate the chakras through these notes, the two most widely used types being Tibetan or crystal singing bowls. Made from different mediums, Tibetan singing bowls are composed of five to seven precious metals, while crystal bowls are made from crushed and heated quartz crystals.[20] You will harness these vibrations as you learn to sing like a yogi in chapter 10, utilizing seed mantras to plant expansion and growth in each of these areas.

Chakra aspect number five is the symbol of an animal, representative of previous evolution. Next is the sixth aspect of insects and divine beings, representing higher consciousness.[21] Neither the fifth nor sixth aspect are used in-depth in Kundalini, though they are actively used in many other lineages.

In Kundalini, we focus on the color and mantra associated with each chakra to activate and harness its unique energy. These two chakra components may be utilized anytime, even if you are not in the middle of a traditional Kundalini practice. Envisioning the chakra's color or mentally chanting the mantra while focusing your mind's eye on the chakra's location will amplify its activatation. The power of the chakras is available to us at all times.

The Seven Chakras

As we begin our in-depth understanding of the chakra system, it is important to mention that the chakras stack seamlessly on top of one another. Traditionally, this stacking is visually shown from the front of the body, with images of circles aligning down the centerline from the crown to the sacrum. A small coil will be located below the lowest chakra if you happen upon a visualization that incorporates Kundalini energy into the equation. The coil, representative of one's Kundalini, is rarely depicted in images—one of the many reasons even the most seasoned Western yogis have never heard of Kundalini.

Minus contextualization, one might assume the chakras line up down the center without understanding where they reside in the body. When the chakras' placement is viewed from the side, you will notice that the system perfectly follows the spine's curva-

---

20. "How Tibetan Singing Bowls Affect Our Body?"; "Feng Shui Use of Crystal Bowls."

21. Satyananda Saraswati, *Kundalini Tantra*, 116.

ture. Here one can begin to connect the intellect behind the science of these locations with spiritual leaders' teachings. The key to unlocking Kundalini energy starts with the alignment of the spine.

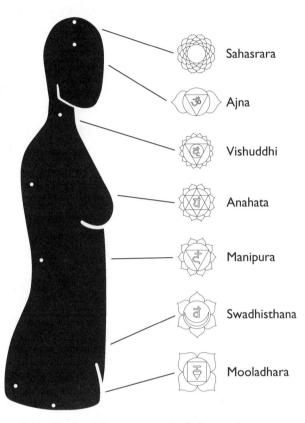

Chakras from the Side

The chakra system is numbered one through seven, with each number escalating from the bottom up. From this side view, notice that chakras one (the root) through six (the third eye) form an interconnected loop of energy within the body. Through the loop of these two energy points, we recirculate the energy of our Kundalini practice within the body. Most meditative Kundalini exercises are performed in a seated position with both legs crossed. Here, too, do we bend the body back into itself so that the energy we cultivate recirculates internally.

Ajna (Third Eye)

There is debate about whether the root chakra or the third eye chakra is the first chakra. In Kundalini, we begin with the third eye. We start here because Kundalini works with intense yet subtle energy. The ajna chakra is worked with and activated first because this is the place of intuition. As you activate the third eye, you strive to approach each situation with a clear mind and heart in the healthiest way possible, processing difficult emotions through reason and understanding, regardless of how and why these emotions surface. Before you strive to awaken the other chakras and move into a space of igniting your Kundalini energy, focus your attention on your mind. As you purify the brain, you make way for all other blockages to be released and processed calmly and effectively, allowing old residue to move out of the body.

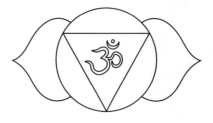

Ajna Symbol

The ajna, or third eye chakra, is where the three most important nadis—the ida, pingala, and sushumna—merge into one, forming higher consciousness as they extend to the crown. Commonly referred to as "the eye of intuition," the third eye is said to be the command center where the inner guru is accessed.[22] Located just above the eyebrows and in alignment with the body's centerline, close your eyes to access this chakra, rolling the eyes up and back, focusing the gaze internally on this location. It might feel as if you are gazing into a *Shoonya*, or void, and it is not uncommon to see darkness as if staring into the vacuum of space.[23] This chakra's location is the doorway through which we enter other dimensions.

Within the symbol of ajna, its two-petaled lotus houses a perfect circle. This circle symbolizes the void, or Shoonya, mentioned above. Within the circle, an inverted triangle represents Shakti, your creativity and manifestation source. Similar to the shape of a

---

22. Satyananda Saraswati, *Kundalini Tantra*, 129.

23. Satyananda Saraswati, *Kundalini Tantra*, 129.

woman's womb, the inverted triangle is diagrammatically used to illustrate the feminine in many lineages. Here this triangle represents the divine feminine at the ajna chakra. Within the void of space, we find divine feminine energy, activated by the sound of OM. OM, located within the center of the symbol, is the seed mantra associated with this chakra. Lastly, indigo's color represents the third eye, allowing us to call forth its energy in our environment with the clothes we wear and the foods we eat.

Mooladhara (Root Chakra)

To close the energy loop, we move next to the mooladhara, or root chakra. In Sanskrit, *moola* translates to root or foundation, the physical location of this foundational chakra.[24] This location is described as the base of all manifestations, both within us and throughout the world. Even in Kundalini, where we address the ajna chakra first, the mooladhara is identified as the first chakra, located directly above one's Kundalini energy. Kundalini energy is also referred to as Kundalini Shakti. As explained in the previous section, Shakti, the divine feminine, is the source of creativity. This energy lies dormant within us until we are capable of awakening its power.

The mooladhara is the starting point for all three of the essential nadis. It is the base from which the ida, pingala, and sushumna originate. It is here that all three of these nadis begin their ascent up the spinal column. Ida, the feminine, represents mental force. Pingala, the masculine, represents vital force. And sushumna, found in the center, represents spiritual force.[25]

The location of the mooladhara is slightly different in the male and female bodies, as the anatomy with which we enter the world varies. Foundational sitting positions are tailored separately to those with male reproductive organs and those with female reproductive organs. Using the following mechanisms, yogis can adjust their positioning slightly to ensure the correct connection to the root chakra. For those born with male reproductive organs, the mooladhara is located somewhat inside the perineum. In a body born with female reproductive organs, the location of the mooladhara is found posterior, near the backside of the cervix.[26] In both male and female bodies, the Brahma Granthi, the knot of the Brahma, is said to be the vestigial gland's location at the mooladhara. This

---

24. Satyananda Saraswati, *Kundalini Tantra*, 137.

25. Satyananda Saraswati, *Kundalini Tantra*, 140.

26. Satyananda Saraswati, *Kundalini Tantra*, 138.

"knot," when held tight, blocks Kundalini energy from ascending. When this knot is unraveled through the activation of this region, your Kundalini Shakti is free to release, moving up the sushumna nadi through the chakras.

The location of the root chakra in the vicinity of the genital region has sparked discussions surrounding Kundalini Shakti energy as unholy. However, the yogic description of this energy takes a different approach. A person's sexual center is the birthplace of creation—quite literally! The sexual center is capable of creating and birthing another human. This energy of conception and the birthing of something new—whether it be ideas, emotions, events, or consciousness—is what Kundalini energy represents. Passing through this solid foundation, the root of all creativity further embodies these qualities.

The four-petaled lotus of the mooladhara is shown with deep crimson or red petals. The square found within represents the element of earth, geometrically illustrating the foundational aspect of this chakra. The practice of *grounding* refers to walking barefoot on the ground, reconnecting with nature's foundational stability beneath the feet. Many images of the mooladhara also show the earth element supported by an elephant with seven trunks. As the largest land animal, an elephant represents strength and solidity. The seven trunks represent the seven minerals, another homage to the grounding elements of this chakra. Just as in the ajna chakra, the inverted pyramid symbolizing the Shakti creative energy is located above the elephant's back. Lastly, the seed mantra Lam is found in the center, denoting the sound vocalized to invoke this chakra's energy.

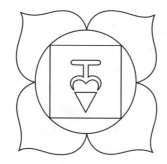

Mooladhara Symbol

Just below the mooladhara is the resting place of Kundalini energy, illustrated as a serpent coiled three and a half times. The opening of the root chakra clears the way for the Kundalini energy to begin ascension. Before we proceed to the next chakra, it is essential to note that if you awaken the mooladhara, this does not guarantee that Kundalini energy will rise. Even if you awaken your Kundalini energy, there is a possibility it may begin to recede and become dormant again. Just as we are continually balancing the body's masculine and feminine, riding the waves of emotion, this energy undulates up and down. To continue forward and be neither complacent nor stagnant, we actively commit to uncovering and rediscovering ourselves in accordance with the ups and downs of life. We do so with the intent of awakening our Kundalini energy, coaxing it upward on its path of ascension.

Swadhisthana (Sacral Chakra)

The swadhisthana, or sacral chakra, is located at the coccyx or tailbone level, the small boney knob above the anus.[27] Located close to the mooladhara, the swadhisthana was once thought to be the location of one's Kundalini energy. The story goes that this energy, which was once located in the sacral chakra, fell, and now resides just below the mooladhara. Because of Kundalini energy's connection to swadhisthana, which was never fully broken, this region of the body and its energy is still considered crucial for a Kundalini awakening.

Correlating to the body's reproductive and urinary systems, the nerves connecting to your sex organs and urethra track are directly impacted by this region's energetic work.[28] This six-petaled lotus boasts the color orange. When you embrace this color by eating foods such as pumpkins, oranges, and carrots, you support your body in awakening this location's energy. The location of this chakra is also associated with Rakini, the goddess of the vegetable kingdom.[29] Due to this connection, the swadhisthana chakra is closely linked to the vegetable world. Eating predominantly fruits and vegetables aids the body throughout one's Kundalini awakening.

The sense of taste is associated with the sacral chakra. In the yogic tradition, two other senses correlate to the swadhisthana—*jnanendriyas*, the senses of knowledge, and *karmendriyas*, the sense of action. Jnanendriyas are also associated with the tongue, just as karmendriyas are associated with the sexual organs.[30] Each connects back to this region's overarching energy of sexual function or desire and the connection to food. Should you

---

27. Satyananda Saraswati, *Kundalini Tantra*, 147.

28. Satyananda Saraswati, *Kundalini Tantra*, 146.

29. Satyananda Saraswati, *Kundalini Tantra*, 147.

30. Satyananda Saraswati, *Kundalini Tantra*, 147.

wish to combat an unhealthy relationship with food or an inability to control your sexual desires, you can perform pranic exercises to move the energy through and out of this area intentionally.

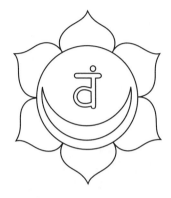

Swadhisthana Symbol

Also said to be housed in this region is the unconscious.[31] In the teachings of tantra, every perception we experience becomes stored in our subconscious. In other words, every encounter, face, word, image, smell, sight, and sound are cataloged somewhere in our psyche. Our unconscious brain moves through our life events, tying our experiences' physical components to our emotions. There are thousands of unconscious thoughts running in the background for every conscious association. We unlock these suppressed memories and emotions as we activate the sacral chakra. It is not uncommon for a flood of feelings to bubble to the surface as these unconscious memories rise to the conscious brain. Following the ancient yogic texts, we are instructed never to presume our subconscious is inactive. Rather, we must understand that the subconscious is in fact the rudder guiding the direction of our proverbial ship. It is with this knowledge that we actively bring the unconscious to the forefront—into our consciousness—to heal.

Manipura (Solar Plexus Chakra)

Directly above the swadhisthana lives the manipura, or solar plexus chakra. Displayed as a ten-petaled lotus, this chakra holds the power of the sun. Linked directly to willpower and energy, think of this location as the energy center from which your physical power

---

31. Satyananda Saraswati, *Kundalini Tantra*, 148.

originates. It is no coincidence that this location is linked to digestive fire. This area, directly behind the navel, is where your digestive system processes the life-giving food you eat. The sun's heat, similar to the heat of a roaring fire, provides us with the ability to assimilate nutrients into life-giving nourishment.

Swadhisthana, the location of Rakini, the goddess of vegetables, embodies the benefits of a vegetarian diet. In contrast, a strong manipura, the area of digestive fire, accentuates the need for voracious energy to process this fuel. One with an active solar plexus chakra is said to have radiant heat—radiance as bright as the sun and energy as intense as a roaring fire. One with low pranic heat to this area is prone to depression, lethargy, and weak physical strength. With a dim digestive fire, the body cannot process nutrients effectively, resulting in the mind's inability to utilize nutrients for healthy brain function. The lack of motivation that follows continues to dim one's light, the energy shining softly like the extinguishing embers of a dying fire instead of a roaring flame.

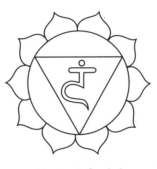

Manipura Symbol

Wearing or surrounding yourself with the color yellow is said to invoke happiness. Yellow, also the color of the solar plexus chakra, emulates the energy of the sun. Like the sun, we rise from the root chakra (the color red) to the sacral chakra (the color orange) to the solar plexus chakra (the color yellow). These colors emulate the full cycle of the rise and fall of the sun each day—a direct connection with the most foundational of nature's functions and the rise and fall of our Kundalini energy.

This chakra is also known as the city of jewels: *mani*, meaning jewel, and *pura*, meaning city. The manipura chakra is the center of Kundalini awakening.[32] If mooladhara is the seat of Kundalini and swadhisthana is its home, then manipura is the location of its

---

32. Satyananda Saraswati, *Kundalini Tantra*, 156.

transformation.[33] For this reason, manipura is considered the most important chakra to awaken Kundalini energy.

Anahata (Heart Chakra)

The Sanskrit word for the heart chakra is *anahata*, meaning "unstruck" or "unbeaten."[34] From your first breath to your last, your heartbeat vibrates throughout your body, your energy field, and the world. As you breathe, purified oxygen moves into your blood vessels, pushed by your prana into your heart. The heart's pulses force this oxygenated blood throughout your system, providing fuel for your body's functions as the blood's metabolic process begins. In yoga, the heart center is located in the spinal column on the inner wall closest to the chest. Also known as *hridayakasha*, this area translates to "space within the heart where purity resides."[35] Your heart center is fed by the purified blood your body circulates. This purification process is amplified through Kundalini's intentional movement of prana.

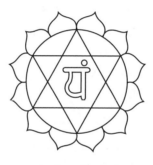

Anahata Symbol

The anahata is the birthplace of heart-centered artistic expressions such as painting, dance, music, and poetry. Here, we learn to tap into our ability to love deeply and express this love creatively. This chakra's symbol of a twelve-petaled lotus houses two intersected

---

33. Satyananda Saraswati, *Kundalini Tantra*, 158.

34. Satyananda Saraswati, *Kundalini Tantra*, 163.

35. Satyananda Saraswati, *Kundalini Tantra*, 163.

triangles, representative of Shiva and Shakti's union.[36] The inverted triangle, the center of creativity, is the divine feminine, Shakti. The upright triangle, consciousness, is the divine masculine, Shiva. The seed mantra found in the center is Yam. You are capable of invoking the energy of an open and expansive heart center as you chant this one-syllable mantra.

The second psychic knot, Vishnu Granthi, is also located at the heart chakra. It is here that emotional attachment becomes tied up in knots; it is the center of deeply felt emotions and experiences. As we progress up the spinal column, activating chakras and untying psychic knots, we do not void ourselves of emotion. As the Vishnu Granthi's untying occurs, emotions settle into balance, no longer holding us hostage under the pendulum swing from one extreme to the other. Just as the symbol of Shakti and Shiva become one in the illustration of the heart chakra, so too do we bring our emotions back to center. Once Kundalini energy reaches the heart chakra, activating each of the lower chakras and associated nadis, and unties the Vishnu Granthi, we no longer have to worry about the possibility of Kundalini energy falling.

Vishuddhi (Throat Chakra)

Vishuddhi, the throat chakra, is also known as the purification center. *Shuddhi* translates from Sanskrit as "purify."[37] When this chakra is activated, the words leaving our mouths are pure, articulate, and concise. The vibration of sound created in the throat shakes off the cobwebs within the body, with each pulse of the vocal cords purifying the body through sound. With the awakening of the throat chakra, you connect your higher consciousness with the other foundational applications of the body's functions, the integral components of the first four chakras. Here we differentiate between higher consciousness and the mind's ramblings. It is the intersection of low-vibrational and high-vibrational thoughts.[38]

---

36. Satyananda Saraswati, *Kundalini Tantra*, 163.

37. Satyananda Saraswati, *Kundalini Tantra*, 173.

38. Satyananda Saraswati, *Kundalini Tantra*, 174.

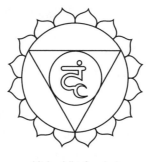

Vishuddhi Symbol

Meditating on the physical location of this chakra's center, combined with visualization of the chakra's blue color and mental recitation of the seed mantra, Ham acts as a triple kick to ignite its energy. As Kundalini energy reaches this chakra, we surrender to the unfolding of life's natural course. This chakra is located at the cervical plexus at the back of the throat pit. Also connected to the thyroid gland situated near the front of the throat, vishuddhi's connection to thyroid function makes the importance of opening this chakra even more critical. The thyroid gland secretes hormones, regulating tasks throughout the body. Through chanting and locking the throat with Jalandhara Bandha, we maintain the strength of our vocal cords as well as the health of our entire body.

The sixteen petals of the lotus symbolizing the throat chakra represent the sixteen nadis that connect at this chakra center. The circle in the middle represents the full moon, and the seed mantra is located within. This is the center where nectar and poison combine. In the tantric texts, a fluid, noted as the nectar of the gods, drips down into the throat. Also called ambrosia (the nectar of the gods), armit (the nectar of immortality), or soma or madya (the divine wine), it is a divine secretion that is also known as the fountain of youth.[39] The concept is that if you can master the duality of life and surrender to life's sacred path, not only will you stop time in its tracks, but you will be capable of turning back the hands of time.

Sahasrara (Crown Chakra)

The visualization of sahasrara, or the crown chakra, has a plethora of lotus petals; one thousand, to be exact. The translation of the Sanskrit word sahasrara is "one thousand."[40]

---

39. Satyananda Saraswati, *Kundalini Tantra*, 176–77.

40. Satyananda Saraswati, *Kundalini Tantra*, 189.

The use of such a large number to categorize this chakra implies the magnitude of its experience. Also described as "infinite," some wonder if the crown chakra was originally named one thousand because it was the most significant and expansive number that could be envisioned. Meditating on its violet color at the chakra's location on the top of the head magnifies this divine connection to higher consciousness.

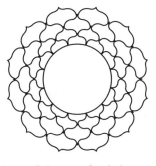

Sahasrara Symbol

Formless and yet with form—everything, and at the same time, nothing—the crown chakra is the portal to infinite possibilities.[41] The location where prana and consciousness merge, it is the peak at which samadhi is reached. Mentioned across most religions, samadhi is enlightenment or nirvana. The moment of communion with the divine is also noted as heaven on earth. Samadhi is only achieved once one's Kundalini energy reaches the crown chakra. It is the location of the void, or Shoonya, spoken of earlier. This is the void of totality, where one transcends the barriers between the earthly plane and the beyond.

We are said to reach this state at the crown chakra because Shiva and Shakti merge. The divine masculine and divine feminine become one, the ida and pingala nadis joining with the sushumna at the crown. All components of a being are working together in perfect harmony, separate but equal, at the same time. Another description of this merge is the death of duality. It is the moment when one no longer sees things as separate, but rather as part of the greater whole.

We have discussed how moving through the chakras via Kundalini awakening is not for the faint of heart. Repressed memories and emotions are brought to the surface to heal as you ascend. The achievement of samadhi, the moment that Kundalini energy reaches sahasrara, is that of pure bliss. It is a place in which you no longer feel pain,

---

41. Satyananda Saraswati, *Kundalini Tantra*, 189.

heartache, longing, or desire. It is the moment when all emotions become one, and you finally experience the vastness of the Universe.

Exercises: Shine Like a Yogi

The following exercises aid in the awakening of your Kundalini energy by igniting your chakra centers. When unblocked, these powerhouses of energy will create transformation and abundance in your life. Utilize the following exercises to bring more alignment into your life.

ᘐ Technique ᘐ
Root Chakra Mini Meditation

Duration: Three minutes.

Posture: Begin upright with a long spine and the chin slightly tucked, in an easy pose or sitting in a chair. Shrug the shoulders up toward the ears, tightly clenching the muscles. Release the contraction, allowing the muscles to soften, with the shoulders rolling down and back. Reach the head's crown up toward the sky, lengthening the spine and releasing compression from the lower back. If there is tightness or pinching in the hips, elevate the hips with a prop such as a meditation pillow, blanket, or block.

Technique: Deepen the breath as the eyes gently close. Roll the eyes up, passing the third eye with the internal gaze, continuing to circle backward. Watch the gaze roll to the back of the head, then the neck's base, then down the spine. The gaze lands at the base of the spinal column, fixed on the mooladhara, the root chakra. As the gaze focuses on the root chakra, see a ball of bright red energy. Begin to internally chant the mantra, syncing the breath to the sound.

Action: Deeply inhale. On the exhale, chant "Lam."

Visualization: As you chant, envision the vibration of this mantra coming from the center of the chakra. Visualize this vibration pulsating the energy of the red ball out from its center. Expanding away from the body with each recitation, the once-small circle slowly grows. This red ball's power becomes more abundant with each breath, extending past the physical body, through the auric body, and beyond. See this energy moving outward horizontally and vertically in all six directions (forward, backward, right, left, above, and below), reconnecting you to Mother Earth.

As you begin to come out of the meditation, start to envision the red light contracting. With each inhale, the circle becomes smaller, bringing clean and clear energy into the body. While still chanting the mantra Lam, visualize all instability and self-limiting beliefs dissolve into the earth below. By the time the red ball returns to its original resting place at the root of the spine, the mantra's chanting is but a whisper. The breath slows and the body softens.

Eventually, when the breath returns to its natural rhythm, allow the body to pause and meditate. When ready, gently open the eyes. You should feel calm, rooted, confident, and prepared to conquer any obstacle.

～ Technique ～
Spinal Flexion

Cautions: Perform on an empty stomach.

Duration: One minute.

Posture: Begin in an easy pose with a straight spine, hands firmly grasping the shins.

Drishti: Eyes gently soften, gaze focusing inward on the third eye.

Mantra: "Sat Nam."

Technique: On the inhale, as the spine presses forward, mentally chant the mantra "Sat." On the exhale, as the belly pulls into the spine, mentally chant the mantra "Nam." The neck remains stationary throughout the movement, unwavering as the spine undulates backward and forward.

Action: On the inhale, flex the spine forward, lifting the chest upward. On the exhale, bend the spine backward, pulling the navel into the spine.

Repetition: Complete the technique for one minute.

Checking the Technique: As you rock, the sit bones remain firmly rooted to the ground. The motion oscillates from the chest to the navel, protruding outward with the chest on the inhale and inward with the navel on the exhale. Allow the shoulders to roll back and down on the inhale, rounding forward on the exhale. Take intentional care to maintain the neck and head's stability as you move.

Benefits: Can increase spinal mobility and aid in the awakening of all chakras.

❦ *Technique* ❧
Spinal Twists

Cautions: Perform on an empty stomach.

Duration: One minute.

Posture: Sit bones rest firmly on the ground, legs bend inward, and heels rest on the pelvic bone in an easy pose. The spine is straight, and the arms are parallel to the ground. The elbows bend, bringing the fingertips to the shoulders.

Mudra: The thumbs touch the back of the shoulders while the remaining four fingertips rest on the front. The palms raise above and away from the shoulders, creating a golf ball–sized gap between the center of the palm and the top of the shoulder.

Drishti: Eyes gently soften, the gaze focusing inward on the third eye.

Mantra: "Sat Nam."

Technique: On the inhale, twist the torso to the left. On the exhale, the torso twists to the right. Take care to lead with the abdomen as you turn instead of driving the motion from the head.

Action: As you twist to the left on the inhale, mentally chant the mantra "Sat." On the exhale, as you turn the body to the right, mentally chant the mantra "Nam." The twisting movement generates from the navel. The head and neck remain straight and in alignment with the spine.

Repetition: Complete the technique for one minute.

Modifications: If you are pregnant or suffering from abdominal restrictions, move gently from left to right, taking care to lubricate the spine without causing pain or discomfort in the abdomen or lower back. This may cause reduction in range of motion, causing the twisting motion to be reduced. Prop yourself on a meditation pillow to alleviate additional pressure on the spine and constriction in the belly.

Checking the Technique: The twisting movement is generated from the abdomen, moving first from the navel, allowing the rest of the body to follow from this movement's propulsion. Make an effort to lengthen the neck and head without straining to maintain a forward-facing position. You will notice that as the abdomen's movement initiates, the body's upper portion naturally follows the action, turning in kind like a ripple effect up your spine. The upper abdomen, chest, shoulders, neck, and head will swing from left to right. The movement initiates from the core, the spine remaining aligned during this side-to-side motion.

Benefits: This technique massages the internal organs, which can increase digestion.

～ *Technique* ～
Sufi Grinds

Cautions: This motion stimulates the lower chakras and might trigger those suffering from sexual abuse or trauma. Move forward cautiously, taking care to pay attention to any emotions that come to the surface while performing this exercise.

Duration: One minute.

Posture: Sit comfortably in an easy pose. Palms facedown, gently resting on the knees.

Mudra: Place the hands on the knees, palms facing downward.

Drishti: Eyes gently soften, the gaze focusing inward on the third eye.

Mantra: "Sat Nam."

Technique: With the body in an easy posture, rotate the body forward in a circular motion, initiating the movement from the navel. As the body moves, the chest will naturally extend forward, following the abdominal muscles' action, contracting backward as the abdomen circles toward the backside of the body.

Action: On the inhale, rotate the body clockwise, initiating the movement from the abdomen. Mentally chant the mantra "Sat" as you inhale and complete the first circle; mentally chant the mantra "Nam" as you circle the second time. The circular motion moves both clockwise and counterclockwise to balance the nervous system and lubricate the spine.

Repetition: Complete the clockwise motion of the technique for thirty seconds, followed by the method's counterclockwise movement for another thirty seconds, bringing the exercise to completion in one minute.

Modifications: Reduce the movement's size to a small circular motion if pregnant or suffering from low back pain. Move with comfort, not to the point of discomfort or pain.

Checking the Technique: As you circle the torso, notice the upper portion of the body follow the circular motion, moving the chest and shoulders as the movement's ripple effect undulates up your spine. This motion is fluid and wavelike. Take special care to remain relaxed in the upper extremities. The neck and head move in the same wavelike motion as the energy moves up through the spine to the crown.

Benefits: Can aid in awakening the lower chakras, which may ignite Kundalini energy, while increasing digestion and reducing lower back pain.

∽ *Technique* ∾
Gyan Chakra Kriya

Duration: Eleven minutes.

Posture: Sit comfortably in an easy pose with a straight spine.

Mudra: Thumb and pointer fingertips press together in Gyan Mudra.

Drishti: Eyes soften to close, focusing on the third eye.

Mantra: "Sat Nam, Sat Nam, Wahe Guru, Wahe Guru."

Pronunciation: "Sat naaam, sat naaam, wha-hay guroo, wha-hay guroo."

Technique: Begin with the fingers in Gyan Mudra, palms facing the ceiling. The hands are at chest height, elbows softly bent, extended away from the body. As the right arm sweeps in front of the body, the palm begins to turn downward, the pointer and thumb finger in Gyan Mudra lowering toward the earth. The right arm crosses the front of the face in an upward diagonal as the wrist continues to turn away from the body. As the fingertips reach the left temple, the palm faces forward, the side of the right pointer finger and thumb now parallel with the earth. As the arm makes its circular sweep over the head's crown, the wrist continues to turn. The right palm faces the ceiling as the arm circles the top of the head. The arm flows over the head and back to its starting position via a diagonal sweeping motion to complete the circle.

As the right arm begins its descent, the left arm begins its ascent in the same diagonal sweeping motion used to create the beginning of the right circle. This time, it begins on the left side of the body and the arm moves up toward the right. The left hand sweeps over the crown of the head, moving back down in diagonal fluid motion. The circular movements are broad and sweeping. Each hand passes across the opposite temple, up and over the center of the crown. The hands alternate so that when the right hand is in front, the left hand is behind, creating a wavelike push and pull between the left and right upper extremities.

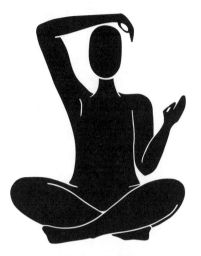

Gyan Chakra Kriya Technique

Action I: As the right hand sweeps over the head, sing the word "Sat." As the left hand sweeps over the head, sing the word "Nam." The right hand sweeps again: "Sat." The left hand sweeps again: "Nam." Next, the right hand sweeps over the head as you sing the word "Wahe." The left hand sweeps over the head as you sing the word "Guru." The right hand sweeps again: "Wahe." The left hand sweeps again: "Guru." The arms alternate over and around the head for ten minutes.

Action II: For the last thirty seconds of the practice, move the arms in their circular motion as quickly as possible.

Action III: Inhale, stretching the arms toward the ceiling, fingers still in Gyan Mudra. Hold your breath at the top, arms locked and spine straight. Exhale as the arms remain stretched toward the ceiling. Repeat: A long inhale, holding the breath at the top, followed by a long exhale, arms still extending up. On the third inhale, the arms remain stretched up. Hold the breath at the top of the inhale and begin twisting the upper body. First, turn left. Then turn right. Do this seven times, with the completion of a left twist and then a right twist counting as one.

As the last twist to the right is completed, bring your body back to the center, exhaling as you softly release the hands to your knees. Meditate.

Checking the Technique: The arms move around the head in a sweeping, wavelike motion. When performed in combination with the mantra's singing, you will feel as if you are flowing through water, softly swaying along with the gestures.

Benefits: Can increase intuition and aid in the release of stored anger. By strengthening and expanding the aura, this technique aids in magnetizing prosperity, calling in opportunities.

Four

Balance Like a Yogi
(Balancing the Masculine
and Feminine Within)

REGARDLESS OF IF YOU were born with male or female anatomy, we each have masculine and feminine energies residing within. Throughout our lives, we pendulum swing between these polarities. Temporarily living in the extreme of either is not a problem; it is when we spent too long at one end of the spectrum or another that we find increased discomfort and disease within our lives.

I spent my early thirties in New York City, living mostly, if not exclusively, in my masculine energy. Not my natural state of equilibrium, this perpetual imbalance wreaked havoc on my body. Ironically, this is also the time in which I discovered Kundalini. Kundalini's methods continually work to bring the masculine and feminine within each of us back into balance. My failing health and perpetual discomfort divinely led me to this art form, and its education allowed me to live in both my masculine and my feminine energies every day with grace and ease.

Masculine and Feminine Energy

Within our bodies reside over 72,000 energy channels known as nadis. Of these, there are three categorized as the most important—the ida, pingala, and sushumna. Ida represents the feminine, pingala represents the masculine, and the sushumna acts as the vehicle for balance between the two. The separate classification of male and female energies is nothing new. Throughout history, most lineages have a way of delineating the masculine and feminine, illustrating the importance of their balance. In ancient Chinese philosophy, feminine energy is known as yin and masculine as yang. Throughout Peru, feminine energy is represented by the metal silver, and the metal gold represents the energy of the masculine. Each variation of this energy ties back to the original symbols of masculinity and femininity, the sun and the moon.

Just as each day illustrates balance with the rise of the sun and the moon, so do we strive to balance these energies within us. Each day we are required to step into our masculine or feminine. Regardless of how you identify, this push and pull of masculinity and femininity feel similar to that of day and night. When in balance, the transition between the two—the rise of the sun bringing the falling of the moon—flows effortlessly. At other times, often due to external factors, we find ourselves moving too far into one extreme or another, causing us to live uncomfortably, even inauthentically, when maintained for too long. It is in these moments that you find yourself in a perpetual state of flight, fight, or freeze. These survival mechanisms of yore were meant to keep us safe, but the stress of the modern world can activate these responses in even the most routine experiences, continually spiking cortisol levels and leading to disease in the body.

Masculine energy is expressed as the container, the structure holding something together, with feminine energy acting as the emotion or flow within that structure. Envision a glass of water. Masculine energy is represented as the glass, while feminine energy is the fluid water within. The glass is firm and encapsulating, clear with an open top. The structure allows the water (or feminine energy) to flow freely, filled up or poured out.

When you swing powerfully toward your masculine, you become more disciplined and task-oriented, hustling toward your goals. As you lean more into your feminine, you flow freely—sometimes too freely—without parameters, focusing on creativity and letting your emotions dictate your life's trajectory. Both sides of the coin are essential. The ability to dip into your masculine and feminine energies at any given moment is a beautiful blessing and resource. With the passage of time, you will swing periodically from ida, feminine energy, to pingala, masculine energy. As situations vary, be it environmental or interpersonal, you have the magic of both sides of the coin available to you. As you begin to dance with these energies, the tools of yogic science are in your back pocket to allow you to transition seamlessly between your masculine and feminine as the situation dictatees. In the following section, we begin to explore how both Kundalini and Mother Nature aid in this dance of balance.

Balancing the Masculine and Feminine with Nature

Throughout history the sun has represented masculine energy. In ancient Greece the name of the sun god was Apollo. His name was Sol during Roman rule and Ra in ancient Egypt. Each of these deities was represented in a masculine form. In Hindu mythology, Shiva is the divine masculine, the complementary counterpart of Shakti, the divine feminine. Taking the symbolic representation of masculinity into the day-to-day, we look to the sun to reenergize the masculine within us. When you feel your emotions start to take over or feel out of control, step outside and allow the sun to shine down on your face. Look to nature to rebalance you in those moments by allowing the sun to provide you with the container in which your emotions may ebb and flow freely.

With 60 percent of the human body made up of water, it is no wonder we feel the ebb and flow of these emotions so profoundly.[42] Emotional intelligence is a crucial component to evolution and survival. Here we also turn to nature to flow with and provide enhancement of this feminine energy. Access to a body of water, particularly a body of water in motion, helps us process emotion and tap into feminine energy. Proximity to the ocean or a running stream may not be accessible to all, but you may still harness these energies by listening to the sounds of waves or rainfall. Looking at a picture or video where water is in motion will also have a similar effect. If you dive too deeply into your masculine, gain a boost by running a bath or taking a hot shower. While lingering under the water's stream, allow the stress and rigidity to gently melt from your energy field, enabling feminine energy to wash over you.

The Left and the Right of It

As you move toward balancing the divine male and female energies within you, begin to pay close attention to your body's left and right sides. The right side represents your masculine energy, and the left side of the body represents your feminine. Through Kundalini's techniques, we work to bring the body's right and left sides into a harmonious union, allowing the energy within to flow freely, creating room for Kundalini energy to awaken. It's essential to keep track of your body and which state it is in at any given moment.

---

42. "The Water in You: Water and the Human Body."

Let's begin with a physical check-in to determine which side of your body is currently dominant.

Prana and Your Masculine and Feminine Energies

Place the backside of your hand just above your lip, directly below your nose. Here you will feel the breath coming out of one or both of your nostrils. As you breathe, which nostril is dominant, the right or the left? Throughout the day, nostril dominance alternates depending on your mental and physical state. As an example, if your right nostril is dominant, your body is craving nourishment, most likely in the form of food. If your left nostril is dominant, your body is tired or sleepy, in need of rest and rejuvenation.

Diving into the teachings of Kundalini, the left nostril, the ida nadi, and the feminine energy within us is represented by the moon. It therefore makes sense that if your left nostril is dominant, your body might be sleepy, ready to settle in for the night under the glow of the moon. In the inverse, the right side of the body corresponds with the pingala nadi and the sun. During the day's waking hours, we need food to fuel masculine energy; it helps with the body's ability to get up and go.

Once you begin to connect the dots between the symbols and energies, it becomes clear how your current mental, emotional, and physical states are continually giving you clues about your health and well-being. Check in with yourself and determine if these yogic theories ring true. Is your body hungry or sleepy, and are those primal cravings in alignment with your dominant nostril?

Discerning the Left and the Right

A few years ago, my closest girlfriends from college and I traveled to Charleston, South Carolina, for a long weekend. Four of us arrived a night early, and as we entered our hotel room for the evening, we began the important discussion of what side of the bed we sleep on. In unison, we each exclaimed, "The left!"—a task not easily accomplished with four people and only two beds. Looking at my girlfriends and the perplexed expressions on each of our faces, I felt called to ask, "Wait, what do you consider the left? Do you mean the left side of the bed when you are lying down, or do you mean the left side of the bed when you are standing in front of it?" To our merriment and a roar of laughter, two of us were referring to the bed's left side as it related to lying down. The other two referred to the bed's left side when standing at the bed's foot.

This is a silly yet jovial illustration of how differently each of our minds absorbs and processes information. To avoid any further confusion, the right side of the body, the masculine, the pingala nadi, refers to the half of the body that contains your right hand. The feminine, the ida nadi, is the side of the body where your left hand resides. This simple dialogue surrounding the body's right and left sides reminds us that in yoga, we must first go inward. Check in with yourself first, taking your right and left cues from your body's knowledge, to access the inherent divine wisdom residing within.

Nadis

Within the body reside more than 72,000 energy points called nadis. This energy's ability to flow freely and uninhibited affects both mental and physical health. This energy framework connects along the midline of the body, crossing at the centerline of each chakra. If the chakras form the trunk of a tree, the nadis are the thousands of branches extending from its core, and Kundalini energy is represented by the roots. By aligning the chakra system, you aid in activating the full nadi network that extends from this core.

Each nadi crosses in the midline of your body through the energy hubs of the chakras. Every nadi does not pass through each chakra, but at least one chakra is connected to every nadi. When you intentionally perform exercises to ignite the root chakra, you are also activating each nadi that intersects this meridian. The ripple effect of balance you feel as this chakra activates extends through your being, with each illuminated nadi pulsating its energy outward to the far corners of your body.

Ida

In Hindu culture, the ida nadi represents feminine energy and the goddess Shakti. Shakti is the Hindu deity of the divine feminine. She is the personification of creativity, and her name in Sanskrit means power or energy.[43] She is the natural balance of the male deity Shiva, who represents the divine masculine, just as ida is the natural balance to pingala.

The ida nadi is also directly related to the moon and its cooling energy. The moon shines brightest during darkness after the sun has set. Also associated with water, the moon's strength controls the tides and represents a more fluid and undulating nature.

---

43. *Encyclopaedia Britannica Online*, s.v. "Shakti," accessed March 9, 2021, https://www.britannica.com/topic/Shakti-Hindu-deity.

This nadi's energy lends itself to the present moment, focusing more on riding the waves of an experience with grace rather than actively moving toward the future.

Your ida is the place where you store information. This energy is one of receiving. Here you take in information, keeping it for later use. The minus sign also represents this calm energy of receiving. By pulling back on your physical activity, you seamlessly receive the information in your surrounding environment.

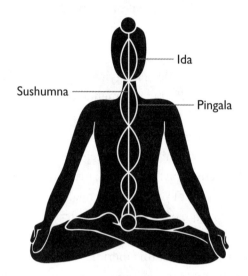

Ida, Pingala, Sushumna

The moments before the sun rises and sets—i.e., the moments before and after the moon takes center stage—are the ideal times of day to balance the masculine and feminine energies. The best time to bring these energies back into alignment are the hours before sunrise and sunset, from 4:00 to 6:00 a.m. or from 6:00 to 7:00 p.m. Take into account slight variations in time due to the changing seasons.

In summary, ida represents the moon, the feminine, the left nostril, and cooling energy.

Pingala

The pingala represents masculine energy, also designated as Shiva. In Hindu culture, Shiva represents the divine masculine. As Shakti's natural balance, he is the yang to her yin. Like the pingala nadi, Shiva represents the sun and the active and heating side of your being. This masculine energy is considered active and fast. Just as every plant gains its fuel by the power of the sun, so too are we driven by the power of the pingala nadi's masculine energy.

Furthering the analogy, in many cultures, the metal gold is associated with the masculine, just as silver is associated with the feminine, with gold representing the masculine energy of the sun and silver representing the feminine energy of the moon. In many traditional marriage ceremonies from India to Peru, the combination of the metals gold and silver in wedding rings is used to symbolize the joining of the masculine and feminine.[44]

Your pingala energy, associated with the right side of the body, is one of processing. This is where your awareness is alert, processing information as you experience it. This processing energy is also represented by the plus sign, depicting this nadi's forward-moving active motion. In the effort to balance this nadi's energy with ida's energy, when meditating early in the morning, it is best to do so under the guidance of another person. When the pingala's fast-paced energy slows as the sun sets, the evening meditation time (somewhere around dusk) is best done alone, preparing the body for the quiet rest and repair of the moon's energy.

In summary, pingala represents the sun, the masculine, the right nostril, and heating energy.

Sushumna

Kundalini practice aims to redirect the prana, or lifeforce energy, into the sushumna nadi to achieve a spiritual awakening. The centermost nadi—and arguably the most important—the sushumna nadi runs up the spinal column interacting with more than 72,000 nadis and the seven chakras. This nadi is neither masculine nor feminine, as it is the balance of both.

The pingala is associated with the phrase "I want" and the aggressive, go-getter action associated with powering forward, actively pursuing goals and dreams. The ida is associated with the phrase "I don't want" and the ability to neither push nor pull, but instead remain in the present moment. This is the energy of acceptance. When both of these nadis are balanced, all paths are cleared within the body, allowing you to dip into both energies simultaneously.

If the ida, the feminine, and pingala, the masculine, are fighting for control, neither will want to abandon their position and will therefore require a trusted, neutral party to

---

44. "Silver Gallery."

balance the scales. This neutral party is the sushumna nadi, the judge. When your brain is tired of battling with itself, continuously asking opposing questions like *Should I do this, or should I do that?*, there comes a point when your brain, exhausted from the struggle, shuts off. This moment when you get tired of fighting and your mind stops thinking is when the sushumna nadi begins to flow. This energy moves from the bottommost chakra up toward the crown, flowing like a river. If your spine is straight, this energy flows more rapidly, igniting more than 72,000 nadis and the seven chakras as it moves. If your body's power was controlled via a dial, turning it to the left, toward the ida, would slow down this flow. Turning it to the right, the pingala would speed it up. Turning it to the center, toward the sushumna, would create a perfect balance.

Chakras and the Nadis

The practices executed in the building steps of our Kundalini practice work to realign and balance the chakras. When we realign our bodies, releasing stagnation and blocks, we allow them to move more freely. As we continue to unbind and open up the pathways of the nadis, uninhibited energy begins to flow.

Much like the stinging sensation experienced when you have a pinched nerve, when the body is out of alignment, you are pinching hundreds to thousands of nadis. When these nadis are pinched or contorted in a way that causes your energy to cease flowing, you lose this transfer of energy within your body. Much like the tingling sensation felt when a leg "falls asleep," so too does much of the body "go to sleep" with the lack of information from their supplying nadis.

Every nadi intersects at least one of the seven chakras. Each of these chakras acts as a junction point for the nadis, much like a train station creates an intersecting hub for a railway. Chakras act as powerhouses, amplifying and supplying the energy of the nadis to all corners of the body. The three most important nadis, the ida, pingala, and sushumna, intersect at all seven chakras. They hold within them the energy of each of these powerhouses, as well as the vibrational energy of every other nadi they intersect. With the chakras activated by all three of these nadis, it is easy to see why they are deemed the three most important. Through their interactions, each chakra's energy is activated. When either the ida, the feminine nadi, or the pingala, the masculine nadi, is disproportionate, the ability for energy to flow freely up the sushumna nadi is blocked.

By working to balance the masculine and feminine within each of us, we realign the body, which realigns the chakras. With each of these chakras stacked seamlessly on top of one another, you can create a clear path for prana to flow up the sushumna nadi toward enlightenment. There will continue to be hurdles pushing each of us out of alignment, as is natural due to the external pressures of modern life. Still, through the daily practice of Kundalini, we work to unblock and clear these hurdles continually.

Through the dedication of a daily practice, the ability to bring your body, chakras, and nadis back to center occurs with greater ease. As the chakras and nadis become balanced, you pave the way for them to be activated. Just as you could not speak if your throat closed, the chakras cannot be activated if they are blocked. It is through continual realignment and unblocking that you make way for your Kundalini energy to rise.

Kundalini Energy

Kundalini derives from the Sanskrit words *kunda*, meaning pit, deep, or cavity, and *kundal*, meaning coil. Kundalini energy is said to lie dormant at the base of the spine, coiled three and a half times. Represented as a snake, images of Kundalini awakening show the snake uncoiling and slithering up the sushumna nadi, through the chakras and toward the crown. Lying dormant just below the mooladahara chakra, you can find this energy's location by placing three fingers below your belly button. Half a centimeter above your third finger is the site of your Kundalini energy.

Awakening Kundalini with the Chakras

To awaken your Kundalini energy, you are instructed to begin at the third eye chakra instead of the root chakra. We focus our energy on the sixth chakra because this is the location of intuition. Through activated intelligence, you are capable of directing this energy—and yourself. If we were to begin at the root, activating the mooladhara first, the body would start to release sex hormones, as this is the location of sexuality and desire. Without the ajna chakra's intelligence, we would have yet to awaken the awareness needed to redirect this energy toward its positive attributes. This energy could turn from creative to destructive if your intuition is blocked, as it could be directed away from that of your highest and best self.

After the ajna chakra is opened, we turn our attention to awakening the other first chakra, the mooladhara. Your Kundalini energy lies dormant directly below this chakra, making it the next step in unblocking for it to rise. As discussed, the mooladhara is your sexual energy's location, but it is also the location of creativity and rebirth. Just as your sexual energy may be used to create new life, so too can this energy be used to develop new ideas, thoughts, and ways of being. With such powerful energy in this region, this area is noted as the hardest to control. Many of our strongest emotions are held in this portion of the body, making this second unblocking one of the seven's most intense.

The Symbol of Kundalini Rising

The representation of the rising of Kundalini energy is found throughout history. The most recognizable of these representations is the caduceus. The ancient Greeks used this symbol as the representation of Hermes's staff. Also adopted by Hermes Trismegistus in Greco-Egyptian mythology, this staff later became the symbol of modern medicine. The caduceus is often misused in contemporary medicine, particularly in the United States, because it is confused with the rod of Asclepius. In Greek mythology, the rod of Asclepius was wielded by the Greek god Asclepius, who was associated with medicine and healing. Regardless of the mix-up, when you see the modern-day use of a caduceus in healthcare organizations, you are looking at a mirror representation of a Kundalini rising.

The staff located in the middle of the symbol is strikingly similar to the sushumna nadi, just as both of the snakes coiling up this center directly mimic the ida and the pingala nadis. You will notice that in most representations of this symbol, the snakes cross precisely five times, with the heads of the snakes meeting at the middle of the staff, at the sixth intersection. The ajna chakra is the sixth chakra and the seat of intuition and the third eye. As discussed previously, the ajna chakra is opened first before we redirect energy toward the mooladhara chakra. Once the third eye is reached, as depicted in a caduceus, the two snakes do not need to cross to activate this chakra because it has already been opened. The uppermost chakra, the crown, is depicted as the top ball of the staff. This chakra does not need activation by the snakes, as it is said to always be open, requiring only the clearing of the other chakras for Kundalini energy to rise.

Exercises: Balance Like a Yogi

The following exercises offer tools to incite the awakening of your Kundalini energy in alignment with the chapter's teachings. Diving into how your masculine and your feminine energy feel within your body will allow you to create greater balance in all areas of your life.

∽ *Technique* ∾
Tapping into Your Masculine Energy

Duration: Eleven minutes.

Through Nature: Walk outside and let the sun radiate on your face. Regardless of the season or temperature, the sun's illumination affects every chain reaction in the body, linked directly to vitamin D's photosynthesis. Unlike other vitamins, vitamin D is synthesized through the skin. Placing your body in the sun for as little as thirty minutes a day strengthens your bones and improves overall bodily function. With this connection to the masculine, you are quite literally building rigid strength.

Exposure to the Summer Sun	*Duration*	*Vitamin D Yield*[45]
Light skin	Thirty minutes	50,000 IU
Tan or medium skin	Thirty minutes	20,000–30,000 IU
Dark skin	Thirty minutes	8,000–10,000 IU

Through Temperature: The use of an infrared sauna is a way to bring the sun's health and energetic benefits to your body's subterranean levels. Far infrared radiation (FIR) is electromagnetic energy imperceivable to the human eye. This energy's radiant heat can penetrate the body up to an inch and a half deep.[46] FIR can invoke detoxification and fat loss. Through a release of toxins, including heavy metals, the body clears itself of impurities on both a cellular and an energetic level.[47]

Infrared radiation, invisible to the eye, is felt as heat, whereas ultraviolet light (UV) can cause sunburn.[48] Today's infrared therapies mimic the FIR light of the sun without the damage of UV light. Harnessing the sun's masculine energy in the form of infrared treatment helps to clean the body of what no longer serves it, providing a pure and strengthened vessel from which to begin again.

---

45. Mead, "Benefits of Sunlight."

46. Healthline Wellness Team, "Infrared Saunas."

47. Myers, "6 Benefits of Infrared Sauna Therapy."

48. Adams, Bero, and Sever, "Planetarium Program."

Through Light Therapy: Red light therapy enhances the mood and cellular mitochondrial function.[49] Harnessing the sun's power decreases skin inflammation and speeds up cell recovery. Visible benefits range from fading scars to reduced inflammation. It is not uncommon for physical therapists and bodyworkers to utilize red light therapy in their sessions because it can speed up wound recovery and muscle repair by causing increased production of ATP. Adenosine triphosphate (ATP), nicknamed the "energy currency of life," provides vital energy for the body's physiological processes.[50] From cell regeneration to muscular contraction, ATP's continual production is paramount to the function of the body.

Not all wavelengths are created equal, but both red light and near infrared (NIR) light have been proven to increase ATP production within the body. This wavelength of red light is seen as the sun rises and falls, when most blue light is removed by nature and red and yellow light predominantly remain.[51] The most effective and cost-efficient technique for harnessing the power of red light therapy is to gaze at the sun during sunrise and/or sunset. As many of us do not have this option—be it due to circumstances such as geography, seasonal change, or the simple fact that most of us spend most of our day indoors—companies now manufacture devices that produce the healing effects that dawn and dusk have on the body.

∾ *Technique* ∾
Tapping into Your Feminine Energy

Duration: Eleven minutes.

Through Nature: Connection to moving water is one of the easiest and most accessible ways to connect to feminine energy. Through exposure to ocean waves, a running stream, a waterfall, or falling water from a showerhead, the undulation of water allows you to tap into the fluidity of your feminine energy. Utilizing Mother Nature as your guidebook, see how your femininity can be both strong and gentle, ever-changing and constant. The oceans' tides, directly influenced by the moon's gravitational pull, express the power of universal femininity. If you don't have access to a natural body of water, you can tap into this energy by listening to waves crashing or viewing images

49. Asprey, "Health Benefits of Red Light Therapy."

50. Scott, "Life's Currency"; "Red Light Therapy Benefits & How It Works."

51. Korenic and Shaw, "Why Is the Sky Blue? Why Are Sunsets Red?"

of water. You can stimulate memories from days at the beach by placing your fingers in some sand. If the running water of a forest speaks powerfully to your soul, listen to the sounds of a babbling brook or walk barefoot in the damp grass to feel dew.

Through Self Care: You can tap into the energy of natural water sources regardless of where you reside. Look no further than a bathroom to tap into this nurturing energy. Taking a hot bath has physical and energetic cleansing properties. As you submerge yourself in water, experience the cleansing powers of this medicine, feeling held, supported, and buoyant in this energy's fluidity. You can access this support in your home or home away from home.

Taking a shower can be an equally meditative experience. Imagine the water washing away negativity. Envision the water cleaning your aura and removing all energy from others clinging to your magnetic field. Your aura, which extends outward from your body, comes into contact with many individuals throughout the day. Regardless of physical contact, proximity alone causes your aura to blend with others. We've each had moments when we've picked up on another's bad mood, feeling their energetic discomfort as our own. Especially if you consider yourself empathic, this transfer of energy may feel as if it is yours, clinging to and remaining with you even when you are alone. Taking a warm, nourishing shower or bath is an excellent way to clear your body of energy that no longer serves you, bringing you back to equilibrium and homeostasis.

Through Drinking Water: Our bodies are composed of 60 percent water. It may seem like a common-sense suggestion, but how many of us drink the suggested amount of water per day? The general recommendation is eight eight-ounce glasses of water each day, though updated research shows that our bodies need more than that. This number varies slightly to compensate for the differences in the male and female bodies. By drinking at or above the recommended amount of daily water intake, you nourish and detoxify while tapping into your nurturing maternal energy.

Suggested Amount of Fluids Per Day [52]			
Male	15.5 cups	3.7 liters	124 ounces
Female	11.5 cups	2.7 liters	92 ounces

---

52. Mayo Clinic Staff, "Water: How Much Should You Drink Every Day?"

↶ *Technique* ↷
Chandra Bhedana Pranayama (Left Nostril Breathing)[53]

Cautions: Chandra Bhedana is a cooling technique; it is not advised during the winter months or when suffering from a cold.

Duration: One minute.

Posture: Sit comfortably in an easy pose with a straight spine. Eyes look forward with the left palm resting gently on the knee.

Mudra: The pointer and middle fingers of the right hand bend in toward the palm while the thumb, ring, and pinky fingers extend straight.

Technique: Place the right thumb in Prana Mudra against the right nostril, blocking the nasal passageway. The pointer and middle finger remain bent while the ring and pinky finger extend away from the nose. The right elbow is parallel with the nose, raised away from the body.

Action I: Gently bring the eyes to close, focusing the internal gaze on the third eye. To prepare, inhale through the left nostril, spine straight, filling the entire body with air. Exhale through the left nostril, releasing all air from the body.

Action II: With the right nostril closed by the thumb, begin the technique with a deep inhalation through the left nostril for a count of four.

Action III: Bring the ring and pinky finger to the left nostril, gently constricting the passageway of air. Hold this breath of retention within the body for a count of four.

Action IV: Release the ring and pinky fingers' constriction, deeply exhaling through the left nostril for a count of four.

Repetition: Repeat inhalation and exhalation through the left nostril for one minute. Meditate.

Checking the Technique: Envision air flowing into the body through the left nostril. This air circulates through the brain's cavities, returning to the left nostril with a final exhalation out of the body.

---

53. *Chandra* = Moon. *Bhedi* = Open/enter.

Benefits: Can reduce heartburn and fever while aiding in relief from anxiety. This technique amplifies feminine energy within the body.

∽ *Technique* ∽
Surya Bhedana Pranayama (Right Nostril Breathing)[54]

Cautions: Surya Bhedana is a heating technique; it is not advised during the summer months or in sweltering climates.

Duration: One minute.

Posture: Sit comfortably in an easy pose with a straight spine. Eyes look forward with the left palm resting gently on the knee.

Mudra: The pointer and middle fingers of the right hand bend in toward the palm while the thumb, ring, and pinky fingers extend straight.

Technique: Place the ring and pinky fingers of Prana Mudra against the left nostril, blocking the nasal passageway. The pointer and middle finger remain bent, while the thumb extends out away from the nose. The right elbow is parallel with the nose, extended away from the body.

Action I: Gently bring the eyes to close, focusing the internal gaze on the third eye. Inhale through the right nostril, spine straight, filling the entire body with air. Exhale through the right nostril, releasing all air from the body.

Action II: With the left nostril closed by the ring and pinky fingers, begin the technique with a deep inhalation through the right nostril for a count of four.

Action III: Bring the thumb to the right nostril, gently constricting the passageway of air. Hold this breath of retention within the body for a count of four.

Action IV: Release the thumb's constriction, deeply exhaling through the right nostril for a count of four.

Repetition: Repeat inhalation and exhalation through the right nostril for one minute. Meditate.

---

54. *Surya* = Sun. *Bhedi* = Open/Enter.

Checking the Technique: Envision air flowing into the body through the right nostril. This air circulates through the brain's cavities, returning to the right nostril with a final exhalation out of the body.

Benefits: Aids in detoxification of the body, which can provide relief from sinus agitation. This technique amplifies masculine energy in the body.

∽ *Technique* ∼◡
Nadi Shodhana Pranayama (Alternate Nostril Breathing)[55]

Cautions: Avoid if suffering from a fever, flu, or cold.

Duration: One minute.

Posture: Sit comfortably in an easy pose with a straight spine. Eyes look forward with the left palm resting gently on the knee.

Mudra: The pointer and middle fingers of the right hand bend in toward the palm while the thumb, ring, and pinky fingers extend straight.

Technique: Place the right thumb against the right nostril, blocking the nasal passageway. The pointer and middle finger remain bent, while the ring and pinky finger extend away from the nose. The right elbow is parallel with the nose, raised away from the body.

Action I: Gently bring the eyes to close, focusing the internal gaze on the third eye. Inhale through the left nostril with a straight spine, filling the entire body with air.

Action II: With the right nostril closed by the thumb, begin the technique with a deep inhalation through the left nostril for a count of four.

Action III: Bring the ring and pinky finger to the left nostril, gently constricting the passageway of air. Hold this breath of retention within the body for a count of four.

Action IV: Release the thumb's constriction, deeply exhaling through the right nostril for a count of four.

Action V: The thumb remains extended away from the body as you inhale through the right nostril for a count of four.

---

55. *Nadi* = Channel or flow. *Shodhana* = Purification.

Action VI: Bring the thumb to the right nostril, gently constricting the passageway of air. Hold this breath of retention within the body for a count of four.

Action VII: Release the ring and pinky fingers' constriction, deeply exhaling through the left nostril for a count of four. This completes one full round.

Repetition: Repeat inhalation and exhalation through the left and right nostrils for one minute. Meditate.

Checking the Technique: Envision the air flowing into the body and through the left nostril, circulating through the brain's cavities and the entire body. Switching the fingers, blocking the left nostril, envision air leaving the body through the right nostril with a final exhalation.

Benefits: This technique aids in the purification of the body, which can provide relief from emotional distress and bring forth mental clarity. This technique can awaken the mind and balance the masculine and feminine energies within the body.

Five

Nourish Like a Yogi
(Nutritional Wisdom of the Yogis)

THROUGH YOGA'S CONTINUED PRACTICE, we purify the body and consequently begin to "wake up" to the reality of the world around us. This increased sensitivity translates to every aspect of life, including the way we nourish our bodies. As you pull away from mass-processed food and consume more fresh fruits and vegetables, you begin to feel these living entities' energy sustain you. As you shed what no longer serves you and synchronize with nature's vibration, your body begins working more harmoniously, performing with greater ease and function.

Alive to Thrive

When you eat food that's alive, you feel alive. Eating a whole foods and plant-based diet allows your body to break down energy efficiently and absorb nutrients. Fresh fruits and vegetables contain prebiotics, probiotics, fiber, and a plethora of amino acids. These nutrient-dense foods are nature's purest form of nutrition. As you consume them, you absorb these energies, fueling your body to maximum capacity.

In most yoga lineages, meat consumption is strictly prohibited. Pulling from the concept that all things contain vibrational energy, by consuming meat, one is thought to absorb the animal's energy, particularly the energy at the moment of its death. The mass farming of livestock in Western cultures amplifies the possibility that the meat consumed has been mass-produced, likely not in the most humane conditions. In contrast, vegetables, even mass-produced ones, are grown and nourished through the power of the sun. When you commit to eating fruits and vegetables that are fresh, local, organic, and in season, you are getting three times the benefits: fed by the warmth of the sun, nourished by Mother Earth, and tended to with caring human hands. Every step of the process is a high-vibrational one, rooted in love, resulting in the most nutrient-dense and delicious food possible.

The Sacred Cows of India

In Hinduism, cows are revered for their generosity and kindness. They are valued for their production of five things: milk, cheese, butter/ghee, urine, and dung. The first three items—milk, cheese, and butter/ghee—are utilized to strengthen and nourish the body. The last two provide fuel to feed the soil and light homes.[56] It is for these five gifts that cows are revered and considered sacred.

Twenty-four out of the twenty-nine states in India currently have varying laws that prohibit the slaughter or sale of cows, though just as not all Indians are yogis, not all Indians are Hindu.[57] Hinduism makes up 79.8 percent of the Indian population, and this majority is generally lumped into one countrywide category, though that is not exclusively the case.[58]

Without an understanding of the history behind why these animals are so revered, one might assume that vegetarianism means veganism. Contrary to popular belief, the consumption of milk, cheese, and butter/ghee is common in even the most devout yogic households. Ghee, believed to have medicinal properties, is an integral component of Ayurveda, and paneer, a widely used cheese, is a staple in many traditional Indian dishes.

Diet for Kundalini Awakening

The food you eat impacts the physical makeup of your body, influencing your mind and demeanor. As Kundalini begins to awaken, the body transforms. This transformation occurs not just in the mind and spirit but also within the digestive tract, making an altered diet necessary. As the body alters, the need for foods to be light and easy to

---

56. Winston, "The 'Splainer.'"

57. Jain, "Ban on Cow Slaughter in 24 Indian States Is Leading to Dead Humans on the Border."

58. Ramos, "What Continent Is India in?"

assimilate becomes paramount. Boiled or cooked foods are suggested, since the breaking down of nutrients begins in the cooking process. This makes them easier to digest and absorb once they enter the body. Animal protein is avoided as it is harder to digest, causing pain and discomfort to the body's already taxed system. Fats and greasy foods slow down and clog the digestive system, adding them to the list of things to avoid.[59]

It is advised to increase your carbohydrate intake as you progress in your Kundalini awakening. Fill up on rice, potatoes, and dal. Carbohydrates provide energy and also help maintain internal body temperature. The reduction of fats and increased carbohydrates may make the diet for a Kundalini awakening seem bland. However, spices play a large role in Indian cooking, and these flavors ensure the food is anything but boring.

The most widely used spices recommended for Kundalini awakening are considered digestives because they aid in the body's digestive process. Aniseed, black pepper, cayenne, cinnamon, cloves, coriander, cumin seeds, green pepper, mustard seed, and turmeric are a great place to begin for any meal. These spices are staples in my pantry. I use them so much that I run out of them regularly. As you experiment with these flavors, note that turmeric must be activated for it to be absorbed in the body. When cooking with turmeric, be sure to add a generous amount of black pepper to activate its healing properties.

Touching again on digestive fire, as Kundalini energy rises and your metabolism slows down, it is even more critical to begin the cooking process in the pan. When you add five or so of these digestion-enhancing spices, you help liberate the enzymes and give your digestive juices a helping hand to break down food quickly. The effective absorption of nutrients is more comfortable when you cook the food first, outside of the body. With warmed food and warming spices, digestive fire ignites. Because you will have a slowed metabolism during the awakening process, eat cooked foods enhanced with digestive spices, heavy on carbohydrates, and light on fat and sugar in order to maintain a healthy internal body temperature. All of these components work together to aid your digestive system. Note: This recommendation is for Kundalini yogis and Kundalini yogis alone, as other yogic branches work the body differently and therefore require different nourishment. For example, bhakti yoga recommends sweets, butter, cheese, and milk because the metabolism will be very

---

59. Satyananda Saraswati, *Kundalini Tantra*, 59.

fast and need additional support.[60] Inversely, karma yoga suggests coffee, raw food, cooked food, and even a little champagne.[61]

Both bhakti and karma yoga boast fast metabolisms as a byproduct of exertion. Therefore, this is a friendly reminder to tap back in to not only your intuition, but your common sense. If you are doing Kundalini yoga every morning and CrossFit every night, strictly following a diet for Kundalini awakening is not the ideal scenario for optimal health. Let your intuition be your guide.

Is your metabolism unbelievably fast? Do you go to the restroom directly after eating? That's an excellent sign of the body working with superior efficiency. Don't switch to a purely Kundalini diet just because the Vedic texts suggest it. If your body is working in superb order, continue on the path you are on. Should you dive deeply into your Kundalini experience, consider slowly adding in the ancient advice described above. As you become more connected to spirituality through this practice, you will find that your body and digestive tract respond in kind.

Fasting

At my Kundalini teaching program in India, my classmates and I were continually taught the importance of fasting, not only as a way to clean and detoxify the body but also as a way to connect with the divine. We will discuss the physical first, for as we begin to move and detoxify the physical body, we make way to detoxify the mental.

Before we come to the spiritual methodology behind fasting, let's first touch on the science backing its benefits. Modern society has embraced intermittent fasting, which has benefits ranging from weight loss to the lowering of cholesterol and blood sugar.[62] Though fasting will inevitably result in weight loss, there are many regenerative benefits to this practice, deeply rooted in traditions based on yogic science.

There is a threshold that is reached in any fasting duration where the action *autophagy* occurs. One of the body's natural cleaning mechanisms, autophagy clears "unnecessary or dysfunctional" cells from the body, allowing healthy new cells to regenerate. This internal process breaks down cellular matter so that it may be used anew. Directly

---

60. Satyananda Saraswati, *Kundalini Tantra*, 62.

61. Satyananda Saraswati, *Kundalini Tantra*, 62.

62. Tello, "Intermittent Fasting."

translated as "self-eating," the internal mechanisms within the body eat, dispose of, and recycle internal components.[63]

The Nobel Assembly at Karolinska Institutet awarded the 2016 Nobel Prize in Physiology or Medicine to Yoshinori Oshumi for his discoveries regarding autophagy mechanisms. Through his research, it is understood that autophagy controls cells' ability to perform the critical tasks of degradation and recycling. This action is highly beneficial for the removal of toxic cells, including precancerous and cancerous cells.

One of my spiritual teachers at the Kundalini teaching program informed us that as soon as he began suffering from any disease, infection, cut, or bruise, the first thing he did was start fasting. His explanation accounted for the fact that the digestive system is one of the body's most energy-consuming functions. Through fasting, he allowed his body to focus on the task at hand. If he cut his finger, the healing time would be shortened by days when he refrained from eating; he had similar results when combating viruses, stomachaches, and most other manners of illness.

My teacher was unknowingly buying into the magic of autophagy. For when an infection enters the body, autophagy begins to eliminate intracellular bacteria and viruses. Damaged proteins and organelles are also destroyed, toting anti-aging properties alongside the ability of the body to heal itself. New research is continually surfacing regarding the benefits of autophagy for health, vitality, and anti-aging. It is no wonder those interested in autophagy range from medical professionals to spiritual leaders.

Introducing Fasting to the Body

As with anything new, it is beneficial to dip your toes into a new experience gently. My teacher suggested beginning by replacing one meal a day with fruit. Should that seem manageable, shift to one day a week consuming fruit for breakfast, lunch, and dinner. As your body adapts to a new normal, you will begin to push your mental and physical limits.

This same teacher stressed the importance of fasting not merely for yogic science philosophy, but also for spiritual connection and the ability to awaken Kundalini energy. He suggested that anyone desiring to awaken their Kundalini should fast for a minimum of one day each week, a full twenty-four hours consuming only water to clean and detoxify

---

63. Zimmerman, "What Is Autophagy?"

the mind, body, and soul. He also suggested that a commitment to this practice should be made for one full year to affect the body physically, energetically, and mentally.

As you embark on your fasting journey, it is essential to note that fasting is not only reserved for food. When you refrain from taking in external stimuli, you also limit energy processing in your body. You could embark on a silence fast, such as in the time-honored tradition of Vipassana. This might also include refraining from social media, television, and negative self-talk. When you fast, you restrict your consumption of people, place, or action to ignite the body into a different reaction.

As Rita Mae Brown wrote, "Insanity is doing the same thing over and over again, but expecting different results." [64] We fast, just as we perform Kundalini, to disrupt patterns. Do something out of your comfort zone to shake up the paradigm, removing all that no longer serves you. Foster change and awaken to a new and sustainable way of showing up in this world.

Eating with the Seasons

Another way to sync the body with the wisdom of nature is to begin to take in energy in the form of locally grown food in alignment with the season. Out-of-season vegetables can be locally and organically grown in a greenhouse during the depths of winter, and should that option be available to you, please enjoy. There is no denying it is a preferable option to the bulk of mass-produced, out-of-season, and out-of-region food consumed by the general population. Greenhouse example aside, focus on consuming the foods Mother Nature has provided when she provides them.

Winter/Colder Climates

In colder climates, generalized as the winter months, there are a plethora of squashes, garlic, leeks, onions, and hearty leafy greens such as kale, spinach, and arugula. There are also plenty of other delicious foods like carrots, beets, and sweet potatoes. Root vegetables shine in the colder months, enriched on a subterranean level by Mother Earth's nutrients. Notice the vibrant colors, natural sweetness, and hearty textures of these delicious options.

Winter vegetables are perfect for roasting, sautéing, or adding to soup. Most of these vegetables are not traditionally eaten raw during colder seasons. Fresh carrots are often

---

64. Sternbenz, "12 Famous Quotes that Always Get Misattributed."

enjoyed year-round, and you might find raw beets in a summer salad, but besides a few stand-alone examples, most winter vegetables are cooked thoroughly before consumption, bringing us to the Ayurvedic principle of digestive fire. Ayurvedic and yogic sciences intersect in multiple arenas, sharing and cross-pollinating many of the same techniques and base principles. Digestive fire is one of the many ways the yogic and Ayurvedic sciences intersect, placing equal emphasis on a principle.

Digestive Fire

The Sanskrit word *agni* means digestive fire. It is an Ayurvedic term to describe the strength of one's digestive system. Compare agni to cooking a meal over an open flame. If the flame is low, food takes longer to prepare. A smoldering campfire rarely brings desired results, where, in contrast, a roaring blaze cooks quickly and efficiently. The campfire analogy illustrates why, in Ayurveda, it is suggested to eat warm or cooked foods in the winter, when exterior temperatures are low, and cooling, raw foods in the summer when external temperatures are highest. As external temperatures rise, use cooling foods to lower your body temperature.

Consume warming, partially cooked foods to ignite your digestive fire in the winter months. The body is already working on overdrive to warm you when it is cold out. With less energy to go around, the digestive system consequently performs at a lower strength. There is a reason warming soups taste so delicious and nourishing when it is cold outside. Not only do you give your digestive system a break by offering it food partially broken down through the cooking process, but by placing warm food within your body, you stoke the digestive fire, warming your system from the inside out.

Summer/Warmer Climates

In warmer climates, known in areas with varying seasonal temperatures as the summer months, when external temperatures spike, most seasonally grown produce is cooling. Cucumbers, melons, celery, tomatoes, peppers, and tomatoes grow bountifully in warmer summer months. These delicious fruits and vegetables also come flush with copious amounts of water, adding hydration to their healing properties. Under the sweltering heat of a summer sun, the body perspires at a higher capacity, requiring more water to run at optimal temperatures. With food being the purest form of medicine, copious amounts of fruits and vegetables provide nutrients and hydration in abundance during heated months. Most of this fuel also produces a cooling effect, allowing the body to reduce and regulate its internal body temperature, even amid the heating effect of digestion.

One would infer that in the colder months of winter, when external and internal body temperatures are at an all-time low, the successful processing of such cooling foods might harm the body's ability to warm and perform efficiently. A smoothie made in the middle of winter consisting of a frozen banana, overly sweet and out of season, would be incredibly challenging for the body to process—especially first thing in the morning on a cold winter's day. It's no wonder people feel sluggish, suffering from stomachaches and weight gain. The yogic practices of yore help the body run at maximum capacity while working in harmony with Mother Earth. Both the land and your internal landscape benefit from honoring the yogis' wisdom: eat in sync with nature.

Exercises: Nourish Like a Yogi

The following techniques aid in nourishing your body like a yogi. Put the lessons of this chapter into practice by healing your body from the inside out with the nourishing power of food.

∾ Technique ∽
Jet Lag Hack

The fastest way to minimize jet lag during travel is to fast. The variation of pressure in airplanes causes excessive expansion and contraction of the abdomen. This air pressure, lower than that at sea level, causes gas to expand.[65] Excess gas builds in the intestines and stomach, causing the stomach to bloat and putting a block in our pipes. When you eat during flights, particularly long flights, the already full abdomen will continue to expand. Gas, a naturally forming byproduct of undigested food, combined with low cabin pressure expansion gives many weary travelers upset stomachs, including excess gas during flight.

Adding in the additional complication of crossing time zones is another variable. As your circadian rhythm fluctuates, sleeping when you would usually be awake and eating while you would typically be sleeping, your internal plumbing further struggles to find its equilibrium. A well-known trick amongst pilots and flight attendants alike is fasting for two to three hours before a flight; drinking water, tea, or black coffee during the flight;

---

65. "Gas and Bloating."

and fueling the body with fiber-rich, plant-based foods upon arrival.[66] This is the fastest way to beat bouts of indigestion and make crossing time zones a breeze.

The body's circadian rhythms are affected by food but superseded by the body's light-dark cycle. When you abstain from digesting during flight, your body looks to the rise and setting of the sun, naturally falling into a feeding rhythm upon arrival. To beat jet lag once and for all, fasting for sixteen hours is recommended, breaking the fast with breakfast in your new location's time zone.[67] This gives the body ample time to reset its master clock. And if you wear a pair of blue light–blocking glasses on your flight, making sure they block both blue and green light to double down on the benefits of the body's light-dark cycle, you may never struggle with jet lag again.

∾ *Technique* ∿
Eating with Your Hands

Throughout much of the Indian subcontinent, it is customary to consume a meal with the hands. The right hand gathers the food, utilizing the fingertips as utensils and scooping the meal into the mouth. The head lowers to receive the food, consuming small portions at a time. The left hand traditionally does not touch the plate; only the right hand is used throughout the meal service. This technique allows you to utilize your natural dexterity to feed your body.

Temperature: As you touch your fingers to your food, you will become astutely aware of the food's temperature. You will immediately know if it is ready for consumption or if you should give it time to cool down. No more burning your tongue!

All Five Senses: Before you enjoy a meal, you become familiar with it through sight, sound, touch, and smell. Eating with your hands allows you to add the sense of touch to the experience before the final act, the fifth sense of taste.

All Five Elements: In the ancient scriptures of the Vedas, the hands are precious organs of action. Connected to all five elements, the thumb links to ether/space, the pointer finger to air, the middle finger to fire, the ring finger to water, and the pinky finger to

---

66. Grant, "Flying Considerations."

67. Bishop, "How to Beat Jet Lag Once and for All."

earth.[68] Eating with the hands stimulates the connection to each of these elements, stirring digestive juices in the stomach.

Connection: Touching the food cultivates intimacy with your meal. Before the food enters your mouth, you feel connected to it, transferring its energy to your body. When food is cooked with love and passion, you begin to feel those energies long before eating. The respect for hard work, craftsmanship, and the skill of growing and preparing your meal is reinforced from the moment you start the dining experience.

Transfer of Healthy Bacteria: As you eat, you transfer good bacteria into your mouth and gut. Like eating yogurt or taking probiotics to add good bacteria to the gut biome, eating with your hands allows additional bacteria to become part of the digestion experience.

Aiding in the Digestion Process: Nerve endings at the tips of the fingers help inform your stomach it is time to begin the digestion process. Feeling your food signals the stomach that it is time to eat. This not only primes the gut to digest, but also turns up other senses like sight and smell, making the entire experience heightened and more enjoyable.[69]

Taste: As explained to me by one of my teachers, when you eat with your hands "the food just tastes better." And to my chagrin, he wasn't wrong. Somehow, eating with my hands did make food taste different in the best way possible. If it is not socially acceptable in your country to eat with your hands but it is acceptable in a country you are visiting, I highly suggest throwing caution to the wind when traveling abroad. The tradition of that visited land has survived hundreds of thousands of years for a reason. By embracing this lineage, you show respect to the area you are traveling, opening your mind and heart to the ways of others. You don't need to understand something fully in order to respect and honor it.

Bonus—For the Kids: As a child, I'm sure I would have loved to eat with my hands. How different would a child's worldview and acceptance of others be if they learned to embrace cultural traditions when eating a new food? Akin to using chopsticks to eat sushi, when eating traditional food from the Indian subcontinent, honor the tradition of enjoying the food using your fingers as utensils. How could this spark a con-

---

68. Please note that these classifications are based on the yogic/Ayurvedic teachings. Other lineages believe in the correlation between the fingers and the elements, but their classifications sometimes vary.

69. Devika, "8 Reasons Why Eating with Hands Is Awesome."

versation surrounding cultural prejudices? Could this be an opportunity to openly discuss emotions about the experience in a safe space? How could that open your heart and the hearts of the next generation to celebrate all races, religions, cultures, genders, socioeconomic statuses, and demographics?

∽ Technique ∾
Sprouting

Sprouting is a quick, simple, and unbelievably cost-effective way to introduce live food into your diet regardless of your physical location. Legumes, nuts, and seeds are some of the easiest things to sprout. Besides ingesting the life force energy of your food as it begins to germinate, sprouting makes these hard-to-digest foods more manageable for your body to break down, resulting in less painful (and embarrassing) gas rumblings in your belly. This also means that in place of fighting against these foods, your body spends the bulk of its energy extracting their nutrients.

Any form of nut, seed, or legume has a protective outer layer strategically adhered for its survival. Through sprouting, you soften this outer shell, opening the floodgates to nutrients previously kept under lock and key. Fiber skyrockets, as do vitamins B and C.[70] Foods that may have previously caused pain during digestion now process through your system quickly and effectively.

Sprouting may also completely change the taste and texture of food. If you have never soaked almonds, I highly recommend it. They swell up beautifully to twice the size of their dried state. The shells slide off, and the taste is so sweet you may never eat an unsoaked almond again.

∽ Technique ∾
Yogi Tea Recipe[71]

Ingredients:
- 15 whole cloves
- 20 whole green cardamom pods crushed to open, exposing the seeds inside
- 20 whole black peppercorns

---

70. Johnston, "Sprouting 101."

71. Kaur Khalsa, *From Vegetables, With Love.*

- 3 sticks of cinnamon

- 8 slices of gingerroot

- ½ tsp mild black tea or 1 black tea bag

- 3 cups milk or milk alternative (I suggest gluten-free oat milk for its thickness and creamy texture)

- Sweetener (optional)

Directions:

1. In a large pot, bring 2 quarts of water to a boil.

2. Once the water is boiling, add all the spices and allow to simmer for 20 minutes.

3. After 20 minutes, add the black tea.

4. Simmer the tea for another 2 minutes.

5. Add sweetener if not using sweetened milk.

6. After the sweetener is dissolved, add the non-dairy milk.

7. Continue to simmer for another 3–5 minutes, incorporating the milk and warming it thoroughly. Be careful not to bring the milk to a boil.

8. To serve, ladle the tea into cups or pour it through a strainer to keep the spices from falling into the cups. Remaining tea can be kept in the refrigerator for up to a week. Enjoy!

Cautions: Do not reheat the entire batch unless you are planning on drinking all of it, because repeated reheating can cause the milk to curdle. Reheat tea in individual portions each time instead.

✑ *Technique* ✑
Stretch Pose

Cautions: Do not perform if pregnant or during the first three days of one's menstrual cycle.

Duration: One minute.

Posture: Lie on your back. Raise the head, neck, shoulders, and legs six inches off the ground as the lower back and bottom remain grounded. The arms reach toward the feet, either alongside the body with palms facing the thighs or with the hands over the thighs, palms facing down.

Mudra: The arms are straight and engaged. The fingers spread away from one another, activated with the palms facing in toward the body.

Drishti: Eyes open, gazing at the toes.

Technique: Lie supine on your back with the gaze toward the ceiling. Raise the head, neck, and shoulders six inches off the ground. As you gaze toward the toes, begin Breath of Fire.

Modifications: This duration of this pose can be gradually increased to seven minutes or more.

Action: Begin with a long, deep inhale. On the exhale, start breathing rapidly with equal lengths on the inhale and exhale. Pull the belly button toward the spine, pressing the back of the spine into the earth as you pump the breath in and out.

Repetition: Repeat Breath of Fire in Stretch Pose for one minute. After one minute, deeply inhale. Release the posture on an exhale.

Checking the Technique: If you feel a strain in your lower back, press your palms and lower back into the ground.

Benefits: Balances the third chakra, aids digestoin, tones the abdominal muscles, and increases willpower, stamina, and projection. Can increase appetite through the stoking of the digestive fire.

∽ *Technique* ∾
Frog Squats

Cautions: Do not perform if pregnant or during the first three days of one's menstrual cycle.

Duration: One minute.

Posture: Come into a squatting position with the heels lifted and the body's weight on the pads of the toes. The knees are turned outward with the belly button tucked in. The arms come directly below the shoulders, the fingertips touching the floor. The toes turn outward, heels touching.

Mudra: The chin remains locked at all times, as does the connection of the fingertips and toes to the floor. The heels stay connected and lifted off the ground throughout the practice.

Technique: Begin in the starting position, taking a long inhale as you stretch the head's crown toward the ceiling. The chest is lifted, and the shoulder blades spread wide with a straight spine. The buttock rises on the inhalation, lifting toward the ceiling as the head's crown lowers to the ground. Fingertips and toes remain rooted on the ground, heels lifted.

Action: As you inhale, the legs straighten, activated through the tips of the toes and arches of the feet with the entirety of the legs straight and engaged. The nose comes to the knees, heels lifted. The sit bones move downward on the exhale, connecting to the heels as the chest, head, and neck lift, returning to the starting position. Move through the inhale and exhale rapidly, with a deep inhale and forceful exhale, lifting and strengthening.

Repetition: Repeat the movement twenty-six times. Lower the heels to the floor on the final exhale, with the feet becoming parallel directly under the hips. Stay bent in a forward fold pose and take three deep breaths. Upon completing the third breath, hold your breath, engage the root lock, and pull the sex organs up and in.

Checking the Technique: As you inhale, the fingertips and toes remain firmly rooted to the ground, while the heels remain connected. As the heels raise, the knees open wide in conjunction with raising the crown of the head. On the inhale, the body will come into a forward fold.

Benefits: Can improve digestion, oxygenate the blood, and realign sexual energy.

Six
Sit Like a Yogi (Alignment and Postures Explained)

AS WE DIVE DEEPER into Kundalini, we will further explore the body's alignment with the introduction of yoga asanas. It is in this chapter that you will take your understanding of chakras, nadis, and Kundalini energy from knowledge to action. As we begin to explore yoga postures, you will learn how they ignite the chakras to help clear blockages from the body. Through this in-depth exploration, you are introduced in more detail to the Kundalini energy lying dormant within each of us.

The Kundalini Experience

Unlike attending a vinyasa class, where the teacher's style heavily influences the flow, a Kundalini yoga experience is more energetically structured. The teacher of your vinyasa class expresses their personality through the stringing together of yoga asanas. The transitions between postures, verbal descriptions, the music playing in the background, and even how they adjust your body as you flow showcase their personality and style. In this yoga lineage, these adjustments are paramount to prevent injury and to help students settle deeply into their practice. However, unlike in a vinyasa class, you will not experience hands-on corrections during Kundalini. This is not because Kundalini teachers aren't concerned with preventing injury; this is because allowing Kundalini students to move through the postures themselves helps keep the process within, making it more personal.

In other lineages, it is not uncommon for yoga teachers to instruct and practice alongside their students. In some Kundalini yoga classes, the teacher will be practicing the techniques with you, both teaching and compounding the exercise's benefits through the addition of their practice. Not all Kundalini teachers practice alongside their students, however. Instead, they instruct with their words, cues, and energetic presence. Regardless of which way they teach, your Kundalini teacher will be located squarely in the front of the room, instructing you as the class progresses.

There are physically taxing exercises in Kundalini, but most of the techniques found in this book begin with the sit bones firmly rested on the ground. One accustomed to the vigorous workouts of a CrossFit or HIIT class may at first find these techniques to be slow, but as the practice builds, you will be amazed at the aches and pains discovered in the most intrinsic regions of the body. Your teacher's personality will also come through in the stringing together of techniques. Different from other yoga forms, Kundalini centers around kriyas, not individual postures or asanas. Kriyas combine various yoga techniques in a specific order for a preset amount of time. Unlike other lineages, what occurs in these kriyas does not change. The length of time practiced may vary slightly—and, if needed, practices can be shortened due to time restrictions or concerns about physical stamina—but the execution will always be identical regardless of where or with whom you practice.

This is one of the many reasons Kundalini can feel overwhelming to newcomers. If you were to enter into a class where everyone appears to know what they are doing, it's probably because they do. Regardless of whether they have entered the studio or learned under the teacher before, they have likely practiced one or more of the kriyas prior as a Kundalini yogi. While this could be intimidating without the foundational knowledge of Kundalini you now possess, let this truth liberate you. Breathe a sigh of relief, and remember that you should not compare your abilities with those of other students. As you continue to practice and a few of the techniques become familiar, the experience of a full-blown Kundalini yoga class will feel both exciting and comforting. What once might have been foreign and scary will now feel slightly more human, achievable by anyone and everyone who has the desire to give it a try.

Building a Solid Foundation

Building a solid foundation is one of the most fundamental components of a yoga practice. Thus far, your yogic tools have been cerebral, intellectualizing the theories and science of Kundalini so that once you begin practicing, the effects of its magic may compound within your body and beyond. When you understand the *why* behind your actions, the execution becomes second nature. A profound analogy for all of life's experiences, when you deeply believe in what you are doing, the *how* becomes fun, even childlike. It is an opportunity to dance with the energies of the Universe to cultivate a life beyond your wildest dreams.

Kundalini's physical practices are rooted in the yogic science of techniques executed in a specific order for an intentional duration. To set ourselves up for success in these executions, in this chapter we will focus on the Kundalini practice's sitting postures. We are beginning to tie together the previous chapters' knowledge, bringing them to actionable steps. The ajna (third eye) and the mooladhara (root) chakras are fundamental in executing all techniques. As we work through the sitting asanas in the exercises that follow, you will understand just how vital the connection is between these two energy points.

Most meditations rooted in Kundalini yoga begin in a sitting posture. Some form of mat, pillow, or block provides stability for these foundational techniques. Providing a separation between the body and the ground allows the energy you create to recirculate within your body instead of escaping below, and it keeps your energy from being affected by Earth's magnetic field. As you sit on your mat, the legs bend inward, redirecting energy to the mooladhara, the root chakra. The hands often rest on the knees, creating another connection point to close the energy loop and redirect the practices' benefits within. With the drishti directed at the third eye, up and in, you further accentuate this energy loop, running the manifestations of your Kundalini practice circularly from the mooladhara to the ajna and back again.

Preparation for the Asanas

The third of the eight limbs of yoga, an asana is a posture of the body. The plural of the word refers to multiple positions, i.e., asanas relate to movements or sequences practiced in succession. If you have attended a yoga class, you have engaged in asana practice. In modern vernacular, a flow is the stringing together of multiple asanas to create an intended result. The focus of this book is mainly on the seated Kundalini yoga postures, initiating most movements from the upper body. Kundalini does boast techniques, such as the ones illustrated earlier in this book, that are not performed in a sitting posture, but the majority of the methods begin firmly rooted on the ground. If you master the asanas in this chapter, you have started the process of creating a foundationally solid Kundalini practice.

The foundational seated asanas—Siddhasana, the preferred posture for those born with male anatomy, and Siddha Yoni Asana, the preferred posture for those born with female anatomy—put pressure on the mooladhara, or root chakra.[72] This pressure provides a catalyst for the release of Kundalini energy. The seated beginning postures, when done correctly, redirect the blood circulation from the pelvic and lower abdominal regions toward the brain. The proper position of the extremities is paramount to redirect the cultivated energy upward through the body instead of allowing it to escape and dissipate into the earth.

Another interpretation of the importance of first implementing asanas in one's practice is the moving of stagnant energy. By performing a few asana movements, you begin to circulate the blood flow and transfer energy from the "stuck" places, creating flow and vibrancy within the body. This flow may be as simple as a few Cat-Cows to lubricate the spine and awaken the chakras. These asanas release kinks from within the body, allowing energy to flow freely. The more vigorous asanas exhaust the body, allowing the mind to quiet and facilitating easier meditation. You will also notice that after most postures, there is a counter pose. This counter posture brings balance to the body, further aligning the bones, joints, and chakras to redirect the energy up the sushumna nadi toward a Kundalini awakening.

Drishti

Many Kundalini exercises will include an instruction for drishti. The drishti, or focused gaze, is a way to bring forth concentrated intention. Often referred to as the "yogic gaze," zooming in on one place or point allows you to block out surrounding sights and sounds, turning your gaze inward. The inward referred to here is that of yourself. By "staring" at one point for an extended time, you streamline your thoughts, bringing your energy back into yourself instead of scattered haphazardly throughout the world.

Every drishti will instruct a specific gaze and focus. Your drishti helps you place parameters on your practice, recentering your thoughts in an otherwise chaotic world. Practicing drishti focus is another way of training your mind. This increased mental

---

72. See Satyananda Saraswati, *Asana Pranayama Mudra Bandha*, 101. This is not a teaching in Kundalini yoga as taught by Yogi Bhajan.

agility allows you to ride the waves of your emotions as you practice, heightening your awareness of these ups and downs, providing you with the skills to observe instead of react when these fluctuations present themselves in everyday life. Different drishtis have different effects.

Posture

To begin the process of awakening, first address your posture. In yoga, just as in life, setting yourself up for success is of the utmost importance. When you put your mind, body, and spirit first, you are setting yourself up for success as you prepare for the day ahead. Aligning this energy with your Kundalini practice, you fine-tune your physical tool, the human body, to dismantle and rebuild the mechanics within. Before we dive into the correct way to sit in a posture, we first address misalignment.

Modern life's habitual movements and patterns have created physical stagnation within the body, making it difficult for many to sit comfortably in the most basic of yoga postures. As an example, excessive screen time perpetuates a forward head posture (FHP). The majority of young people today have their head, neck, and shoulders perpetually curved forward due to excessive screen time. In this posture, the cervical vertebrae move forward, becoming hyperextended. This hyperextension, combined with an inward shoulder curve, creates rounding in the upper back. This rounding results in persistent pain from the shortened muscles in the lower neck. A small tilt of just fifteen degrees forward increases the force on the neck from about ten pounds to twenty-seven pounds. Unaddressed, a forward head posture might extend to forty-five degrees, adding a burden of almost forty extra pounds for the shoulders to carry.[73] This causes a person's body to feel as though it is carrying excess weight due to the skeletal system's misalignment.

When you envision the act of going for a run, it becomes apparent just how significant the head's slight tilt impacts the remainder of the body. How much more difficult would it be to keep a smooth cadence if you were trotting down a path with an additional thirty-five pounds of weight on your shoulders? Not the easiest of tasks, to be sure, made even more complicated as you come to understand how this uneven distribution of the skeletal system affects the entirety of your body. The neck and shoulder pain from the shortening of the muscles in the back of the neck creates persistent pain in this region,

---

73. Admin, "Forward Head Posture."

giving way to a cascade of misalignments that attempt to compensate for this uneven distribution of weight.[74]

As you sit on your meditation pillow, feel the effect of this example by tilting your head forward. The forward head position creates tightness in the lower back as the lower lumbar begins to load from the additional weight. This tightness causes the abdomen and pelvis to tip forward, making the abdomen look potbellied, and the hip joints tighten. The ripple effects continue as the pelvic position causes the hamstrings to tighten and the calves to overwork, which will result in a loss of flexibility and instability in the ankles and feet. If your hips and spine are continually out of alignment, you can feel FHP even as you sit cross-legged on your mat. You might need to prop your hips up on a pillow to reduce the lower lumbar spine loading and relieve the tension in your hips.

This example is used to examine the chain reaction that something as simple as a tilt of the head can have on the entire body. I did not share this for the sake of an anatomy lesson, but instead to illustrate the physical repercussions that can be seen with the naked eye. After too many hours spent staring at a computer screen or a phone, people begin to feel physical pain. Your muscle memory might literally cause your neck and shoulders to ache as you recall the experience. Now imagine the chain reaction that this misalignment causes that you cannot see! With increased loading in your lumbar spine, what nerves are you pinching, and what signals are those nerves sending to your body? How is your digestive system impacted? What about your lungs' ability to operate at full capacity or your heart's ability to beat unencumbered? With each action's resulting alignment or misalignment, you are continually sending signals to your body, physically and energetically.

OPENING YOUR HEART

Stress, strain, and misalignment cause excess fluid to form within the muscles. As this fluid converts to swelling, knots made up of waste product form, restricting movement and causing pain. The act of lengthening your muscles dislodges these stuck toxins, allowing them to begin expulsion from the body. In a yoga practice, you are likely familiar with the lengthening of your larger muscles, like the hamstrings in a forward fold or the quadriceps in a crescent lunge, but when was the last time you thought of lengthening your most important muscle, the heart? The muscles across your chest and back act

---

74. Physiopedia Contributors, "Forward Head Posture."

as an added barrier of protection for your heart. Physically protected by the ribs, the muscles encasing this structure provide additional layers of energetic protection.

If you are suffering from a broken heart, your body's physical reaction closes rank around your heart center. The surface area visible to the world becomes small and concave. Your shoulders round and your chin tucks; your body is beginning to mimic the upper ball of a fetal position as you fold into yourself. As you notice yourself leaning forward, instead of focusing on the pain in the shoulder, neck, and chest, what would happen if you lovingly wrapped your arms around yourself? First, grasping so tightly that you pull the shoulder blades apart, lengthening the muscles across your upper back. Could you stretch so profoundly and hug yourself so tightly that you simultaneously release the toxins of your sorrow from these muscles' depths? Can you hold on tight, not only for a moment, but for several minutes? Relish your touch, curl your chin inward, and embrace your heart with these loving arms. Here you intentionally mimic the nurturing embrace of the fetal position instead of falling victim to it.

As you release the grip from this hug, your neck will lengthen. You grow slightly taller and the surface area of your chest will jut out toward the rest of the world. As your shoulders release and soften, your heart area opens slightly more. The back side of the heart is where we experience the energy exchange from another, the act of receiving love. The heart's front side is where we shine our loving light into the world, the act of giving love. As you hug yourself, you expose more of the back surface, energetically welcoming love from others. When toxins release from the back body's muscles, you clear stagnation, making room for this love to be received. The simple act of hugging yourself removes toxins, physically and energetically. Your heart softens as you give yourself the love you wish to receive.

The End Goal

Once you become acutely aware of how misaligned postures affect your body, you can begin to pay close attention to the subtle energetics of your actions. Kundalini allows you to tap into these resistance areas to move energy. The belief is that the more freely and unencumbered your body moves, the greater your ability to effectively process and express information. This uninhibited mind and body allow you to deeply tap into your spiritual practice, making way for you to reach your highest potential. When you remove physical blocks, you begin to feel the subtleness of the breath. As the breath moves freely throughout the body, you awaken the nadis, igniting your life force energy. With life force energy pumping through your veins, added mudras, mantras, and bandhas in your kriya practice help you achieve pinpointed results. After all of that pinpointed attention—your body in alignment, your breath in sync, and your energy flowing freely throughout your body—pause.

This pause is where the magic happens. It may seem like a lot of work; there are so many steps to sit in meditation and intentionally be one with yourself. The process feels arduous when written in paragraph form, but it is actually quite simple. Kundalini's beauty is that you can achieve life-altering results in just a few short minutes, particularly when you commit to putting your mind, body, and spirit first every day.

Here is an example of a twelve-minute full asana, pranayama, kriya, and meditation practice:

- Minute 1: Tune in

- Minutes 2–3: Three rounds of Cat/Cow

- Minutes 4–6: Alternate Nostril Breathing and Breath of Fire

- Minutes 7–9: Meditation to Heal Addictions

- Minutes 10–12: Silent meditation

- Minute 12: Tune out; close practice

Through each of the lineages of yoga, the exercises are all designed with the same result. Be it a power yoga class with weights, a hip-hop vinyasa flow, or a slow restorative class, each movement is intentionally sequenced to allow the body to release and the mind to soften. In Kundalini yoga, we do breathing exercises, postures, and kriyas so the body is stretched, lengthened, strengthened, and capable of becoming quiet, allowing the voice of the highest and best self to come through and be heard clearly.

Dropping into a meditative state will enable you to reengage with your soul. The noise of the world falls away, and you are able to see things more clearly. I liken it to a bird soaring high in the clouds. You can feel the cool breeze of the air, touch the clouds' majesty with your wings, and feel the bright warmth of the sun on your face, observing the world below with clear and unobstructed eyes. From this vantage point, you see the big picture more clearly. You begin to connect the dots, stringing together the previously fragmented components of your thoughts.

Meditation's goal is not to remove all thoughts from your mind. What meditation allows you to do is observe those thoughts from a bird's-eye view without judgment. You watch the running tape stream across the proverbial picture screen in your mind, allowing your thoughts to come and go. You remove the internal and external floodgates previously holding each of these thoughts and emotions at bay through asanas, pranayama, and kriyas; this is the trick of meditation that so many get confused by when they first begin. You likely settled in for your first "sit" and felt instantly bombarded by the magnitude of thoughts and emotions flooding your mind. It feels overwhelming, stressful, and painstakingly counterproductive.

It's especially confusing when the general misconception surrounding meditation is that the point of meditation is to quiet the mind. As the bombardment of thoughts begins, it can feel like an ocean's wave continually knocking you down: *How can my mind be quiet when everything on my to-do list is waiting for me? Did I turn the oven off? What should I eat for dinner? Why did I just think about my second-grade boyfriend, whom I haven't thought of in twenty years?* With insurmountable evidence that the mind is anything but quiet, how is meditation achievable when you have been told you need to make the dialogue stop? The secret is, you don't. All of those thoughts, every far-fetched one of them, have always been there. They are continually running on a loop in the background. They are the white noise of your life, so consistently present that you don't realize they're there.

This is when the surrender comes. This is when the shoulders finally begin to relax and the tightness behind your eyes softens. You are hit with the realization that there is nothing you need to fix, move, or add on to the ever-mounting list of to-dos. All of those thoughts have been there all along. They will never go away, for as we live and breathe, the beauty of this life is that we experience and interact with new challenges, obstacles, people, places, and emotions every day. It's one of the marvelous things about being alive. You can put down the sword, because you no longer need to fight yourself; instead, embrace yourself as the whole and perfect being you are.

How much better does it feel to know that you no longer have an invisible wall to climb or a boundary within yourself? Thoughts are just thoughts, and emotions are only emotions. They come and go. We experience life-altering highs and mind-numbing lows, yet neither the feelings nor experiences of these extremes is permanent. With the knowledge of this impermanence, embrace your Kundalini practice, welcoming the meditative results it creates, and be conscious of its continual fluctuation. Make friends with the voices in your head; embrace your Kundalini energy and ask it to come forth. For once you befriend your soul, you know the best is yet to come.

The Power of the Pause

Kundalini is arguably the most meditative and spiritual of the yogic lineages. Kundalini focuses on the subtle nuances of the body and mind to achieve balance—balance within yourself, your environment, and your ecosystems. Kundalini was developed from the belief that when we push past our physical, mental, and emotional limitations and over-exert ourselves, we lose the ability to maintain awareness. Its focus is on helping an individual find the right balance between pushing too hard and not pushing enough.

You might find yourself unable to sustain continued focus in the present moment. Your mind may be continually flickering from memories of the past to dreams and worries of the future. This makes it difficult to relish the moments you experience as you experience them. Kundalini yoga teaches us that these experiences, such as the moment you are taking right now to read this very page, are the most important of all—arguably the only moments that matter.

Glenn Turner said, "Worrying is like a rocking chair. It gives you something to do but gets you nowhere." If I could choose one quote to embody the spirit of a modern Kundalini practice, it would be this one. Worrying is rooted in the past and the future. As we sit swaying in a rocking chair, like the one I am ebbing and flowing in as I write these very lines, we find ourselves in continual motion, moving forward and backward. This is the perfect metaphor for the mind because worrying is a constant teeter-totter between the past and the future, one that skips over the present moment entirely. When we worry, the mind begins to stress about something that happened in the past and how it will affect the future. The right and left foot of worry are perfectly straddled, one in front and one behind, bypassing the present moment's stability.

What would happen if we slowed the rocking chair, pausing in the center instead of teetering on the edge? Could your heart rate start to slow as the pace of the rocking begins to soften? Would your breath begin to even out, matching the slower pace of the chair's stride? This is what begins to happen as you cultivate your Kundalini practice. You begin to harness the "power of the pause." The meaning is twofold. We liken the pause to the ability to be fully present in moments as they unfold, and there is also the ability to pause, think, and process before reacting.

Like all yoga, Kundalini teaches that how you show up on your mat or meditation pillow is how you show up in everyday life. Suppose you power through strenuous asanas, forcing and straining during your practice. There is a strong possibility that you find yourself pushing, twisting, and powering through your daily life. The postures, breathwork, mantras, mudras, and kriyas of Kundalini work together to disrupt the patterning of your mental, physical, and emotional loops. Kundalini seeks to edit your internal dialogue, which is continually playing on repeat in the background.

When you push and force, your body responds in kind. In contrast to the aches of sore muscles that are lengthened and strengthened from intentional physical effort, today's "powering through" attitude cultivates chronic pain and misalignment. Continual stress results in the overcompensation of specific muscles while fostering lethargy and potential atrophy in others. Our bodies, like life, work in a carefully orchestrated balance. When you find yourself with external physical misalignment, you will likely also discover that your body's inner workings are off-kilter. We've all experienced days when we felt out of whack, when left seems to be right, up seems to be down, and nothing goes quite according to plan. This is the physical manifestation of your internal misalignment.

As you deepen your connection to your body, mind, and spirit, you begin to become in tune with the interconnectedness of all three. Through Kundalini, you actively work to repair the physical, mental, and spiritual simultaneously. By adjusting your external body into proper alignment, so too do you align the internal. As your organs, bones, and muscles work effortlessly, your heart begins to open. As your heart opens and the energy centers along your spine are activated, the consciousness of your mind is awakened as well. Heightened awareness allows you to begin to make friends with the voices in your head. You come to see your inner self as a friend instead of an enemy to be squashed or ignored. The cycle of alignment continues as kinder internal dialogue dissipates stress, allowing you to remain in symbiotic external alignment because you now live from a higher vibration. Each affirmative action of bringing your heart, body, mind, and spirit back to the center allows them to flow freely. The heart, body, mind, and spirit are uninhibited, unencumbered, and unwavering in their ability to repair themselves, regardless of the adversity.

Kundalini is high-vibration energy. It is energy that shakes up the old paradigm of your psyche. Through your Kundalini practice, you are encouraged to come face-to-face with your demons. Face them, name them, feel them, embrace them, and then let them move. This is a far cry from the New Age rhetoric of "thinking positively" to receive; Kundalini allows you to embrace both sides of yourself. We are each born with light and dark, Shiva and Shakti, masculine and feminine. It is through Kundalini that we learn how to balance this energy effectively. Through Kundalini, you awaken the nadis, unblock the chakras, and allow the source of your highest potential, your Kundalini energy, to flow freely through you.

Exercises: Sit Like a Yogi

Learn how to align your spine and prepare your body for your Kundalini practice. The following techniques will allow you to create a solid foundation to begin your Kundalini journey.

∽ *Technique* ∾
Ardha Padmasana (Half Lotus)[75]

Cautions: Do not perform if suffering from sciatica or experiencing knee pain.

Duration: One minute.

Posture: Begin on the sit bones with the legs extended in front of the body. Bend the right knee, bringing the sole of the right foot against the left inner thigh. Press the right heel against the perineum, creating slight pressure on the mooladhara (root chakra). Bend the left knee, placing the left foot on top of the right thigh. With as little strain or cranking of the left foot as possible, strive to bring the left heel against the lower abdomen. This foot placement connects to the swadhistana (sacral chakra).

Technique: The legs are locked with both knees firmly placed on the ground. The spine is straight.

Modifications: If placing the foot on top of the thigh causes you to strain or crank your foot into place, begin by first placing only the toes, allowing the top of the foot to press against the inner thigh. If you feel strain in your hips, elevate the body by placing a meditation pillow or block under your sacrum. This posture may be performed with either the left or the right foot up.

Checking the Technique: The sit bones press firmly into the ground, mat, or meditation pillow. One heel presses against the pubic bone while the other is pressed against the abdomen.

---

75. *Ardha* = Half. *Padmasana* = Lotus.

Benefits: This technique works to calm the nervous system, which can stimulate digestion, and redirects blood flow from the lower regions of the body upward.

∾ *Technique* ∾
Padmasana (Lotus)

Cautions: Do not perform if suffering from sciatica or experiencing knee pain. This asana should only be performed after the flexibility of the knees has been developed through other asanas.

Duration: One minute.

Posture: Begin on the sit bones with the legs extended in front of the body. Bend the left knee, bringing the top of the foot to the top of the opposite leg's inner thigh. The toes rest against the top of the leg while the upper foot bends, softening across the thigh's upper inside portion. Bend the right knee, crossing the shin over the opposite leg. The underside of the foot faces upward on top of the opposite thigh. With as little strain or cranking of the left foot as possible, strive to bring the left heel against the lower abdomen. The heels of both feet connect to the lower abdomen at the swadhistana (sacral chakra).

Mudra: When used for meditative purposes, this posture is traditionally performed with the backs of the hands on the knees in Chin or Jnana Mudra.

Technique: When the legs are locked, both knees firmly rest on the ground. The spine is straight, and the tailbone is rooted below. This posture may be performed with either the left or the right foot upward, though it is traditionally taught to bring the left leg into the body first and then place the right leg on top.

Modifications: Should the posture feel uncomfortable, alter the legs. Begin again by placing the second leg on the opposite thigh first. If you notice straining in the hips, elevate the body by placing a meditation pillow or block under the sacrum.

Checking the Technique: The soles of the feet are turned up with the heels of the feet pressing against the pubic bone. The pubic bone should be firmly rooted on the ground, allowing for a long spine without pain or strain.

Benefits: This technique can stimulate digestion while redirecting blood flow from the lower regions of the body upward. It provides a heightened meditative experience because the closed loop of energy circulates the energy within the body through all seven chakras.

⟆ *Technique* ↷
Siddhasana (Accomplished Pose for Men)

Cautions: Do not perform if suffering from sciatica or lower back pain caused by the sciatic nerve.

Duration: One minute.

Posture: Begin on the sit bones with the legs extended in front of the body. Bend the right knee, bringing the sole of the right foot against the left inner thigh. Press the right heel against the perineum, creating slight pressure on the mooladhara (root chakra). Bend the left knee, placing the left ankle over the right ankle. The ankle bones touch with the heels on top of one another—the left heel presses against the pubic bone, directly above the genitals. Pull the left toes to the space between the right thigh and calf, and pull the right toes into the area between the left thigh and calf.

Technique: The legs lock with both knees firmly placed on the ground and a straight spine.

Modifications: As you practice this asana, it is helpful to begin with the hips elevated. The use of a rolled blanket, yoga mat, or block to raise the hips releases pressure on the lower back, allowing you to ease into the posture.

Checking the Technique: For the placement of the two heels to be correct, ensure the male genitalia is located directly between them. By grasping the right toes from above or below, pull the right foot up, placing it into the space between the left thigh and calf. The legs should feel locked in place.

Benefits: Can calm the nervous system while redirecting blood flow from the lower regions of the body upward.

⟆ *Technique* ↷
Siddha Yoni Asana (Accomplished Pose for Women)

Cautions: Do not perform if suffering from sciatica or lower back pain caused by the sciatic nerve.

Duration: One minute.

Posture: Begin on the sit bones with the legs extended in front of the body. Bend the right knee, bringing the sole of the right foot against the left inner thigh, the right heel pressing against the labia majora. Bend the left knee, placing the left ankle over the right ankle. The left heel is pressing against the clitoris. The ankle bones touch and the heels stack on top of one another. Pull the left toes to the space between the right thigh and calf, and pull the right toes into the area between the left thigh and calf.

Technique: The legs lock with both knees firmly placed on the ground. The spine is straight.

Modifications: As you practice this asana, it is helpful to begin with the hips elevated. The use of a rolled blanket, yoga mat, or block to lift the hips releases pressure on the lower back, allowing you to ease into the posture.

Checking the Technique: Shimmy the left toes down so they touch (or almost touch) the floor. From above or below, pull the right toes up to the left calf and thigh space. Both the knees and the sit bones touch the ground.

Benefits: Can calm the nervous system while redirecting blood flow from the lower regions of the body upward.

↷ *Technique* ↶
Vajrasana (Thunderbolt)

Cautions: Proceed with caution if suffering from sciatica or experiencing knee pain.

Duration: One minute.

Posture: Begin kneeling on the floor with the knees together. The toes come to touch as the heels separate. The heels graze the side of the hips as the lower portion of the buttocks rests on the inverted triangle made by the feet.

Mudra: Place the hands on the knees, palms facing downward.

Drishti: Eyes gently soften, gaze focusing inward on the third eye.

Technique: The knees and upper thighs press firmly against one another as the head's crown reaches toward the ceiling with a straight spine.

Modifications: A block is a beautiful modification that allows you to bring the ground to you to maintain a long, straight spine. The block situates between the feet at the desired height. The goal of the prop is to allow ease and comfort in the pose while maintaining proper posture. If you begin to feel pain in the thighs, separate the knees slightly and continue.

Checking the Technique: Using the palms, gently grab the calves and roll the flesh away from the body, allowing the body's weight to sit firmly against the pads of the feet and heels. To gain proper spine alignment, begin by rocking the pelvis forward and then backward. As you exaggerate each movement, you strengthen your body awareness, allowing you to find your center alignment or posture of ease more easily.

Benefits: Can strengthen the pelvic floor and increase digestive efficiency.

⌒ *Technique* ⌒
Shoulder Shrugs

Cautions: Perform with less vigor if suffering from neck or shoulder injuries, moving softly through the motion.

Duration: One minute.

Posture: Begin in an easy pose with a straight spine, palms resting on the knees.

Drishti: Eyes gently soften, gaze focusing inward on the third eye.

Mantra: "Sat Nam."

Technique: On the inhale, shrug the shoulders toward the ears. On the exhale, allow the shoulders to fall, releasing the tension in the muscles.

Action: On the inhale, intentionally contract the muscles in the shoulders and neck. As you exhale, feel the tension dissipate as you sigh deeply, releasing the tension in the muscles. As you move through this sequence, mentally chant "Sat" on the inhale and "Nam" on the exhale.

Repetition: Repeat for one minute.

Checking the Technique: As you shrug, actively pull the shoulders toward the ears, executing the motion vertically, intentionally moving in a straight line up and down. The neck remains long, gaze fixed on the third eye, taking care not to tilt the shoulders forward or backward as they move up and down.

Benefits: Increases circulation to the heart, neck, and shoulders. Can release tension in the upper body and increase mobility in the shoulders and neck. Proper alignment of the spine may be achieved once tension in the neck and shoulders is released.

⌯ *Technique* ⌯
Meditation on the White Swan

Duration: Three minutes.

Posture: Sit comfortably in an easy pose.

Mudra: The fingertips curl into the palms while the tips of the thumbs press against one another. Palms face away from the body. The thumbs are in alignment with the nose, and the tips of the thumbs are level with the brow. The thumbs come to rest a few inches in front of the body. Press the tips of the thumbs firmly against one another until the pads turn slightly white. Allow the first joint of the thumb to bend as much as possible; this pressure should be comfortable, not restrictive or from a place of strain or pain.

Drishti: Fix the gaze at the thumbs for a few seconds, mentally imprinting this image so that as you softly close the eyelids, you see the thumbs in your mind's eye.

Mantra: "Sat Nam."

Technique: Raise the arms to shoulder height, bending the forearms inward to bring the hands into the mudra. Focus your gaze on the tips of the thumbs for a few seconds before closing your eyes, envisioning the thumbs in your mind's eye with your eyelids closed.

Action: With the eyes closed, begin taking slow deep breaths while mentally vibrating the mantra "Sat" on the inhale and "Nam" on the exhale.

Repetition: Repeat the technique for three minutes.

Modifications: Elevate the hips on a block or pillow if suffering from knee pain or lower back pain.

Checking the Technique: The arms begin parallel to the ground. The forearms bend inward, connecting the mantra's thumb tips, creating an incomplete heart with the hands.

With the thumb in alignment with the nose and the tips of the thumbs at eyelid height, you will notice a heart form in the negative space of the two hands.

Benefits: Aids in deep relaxation. This is a wonderful kriya to practice before bed for a restful night's sleep.

Seven
Breathe Like a Yogi
(Breathwork to Detoxify and Realign)

WITH THE SITTING POSTURES now firmly rooted in your practice, we can begin harnessing prana, life force energy, to circulate and direct the breath throughout the body. I first learned of the breath's cleansing properties while studying to be a Pilates instructor in my early twenties. Joseph Pilates called the act of breathing the "internal shower," noting that via breathing exercises, we purify our systems from the inside out.[76] We remove impurities from the body through proper breathing, expelling toxins and promoting overall health. The science behind the breath as an internal shower is found in Pilates and across all yogic lineages. Yoga techniques cleanse the body mentally, emotionally, physically, and spiritually through the execution of pranayama, the techniques that move your prana. This paves the path to a Kundalini awakening. The breathing techniques that follow recalibrate your system, remove toxins, and bring life force energy into every cell.

What's in a Breath?

The average person takes approximately 20,000 breaths a day.[77] On the opposite end of the spectrum, it has been documented that the great yogis—the master gurus of the ages—take far fewer breaths, an astonishing seventy to 108 breaths per day. In today's

---

76. Pilates and Miller, *Return to Life Through Contrology*, 8.

77. "How Many Breaths You Take Per Day and Why It Matters."

modern age, this feat sounds virtually impossible. Most of us, myself included, execute what is considered a shallow breath instead of long, deep breaths. When you shallow-breathe, you take short breaths, filling the throat with air. Air enters the top portion of your chest cavity when you do this, reaching only the uppermost part of your lungs. Although this type of breath is satiating enough to keep you alive, it does very little for your overall health, barely scraping the surface of the life-giving properties of your prana. This is especially concerning when you consider that traditional yogic philosophy says that the breath controls the mind. But most of us rarely—if ever—take full deep breaths that fill up the lungs entirely. The average male has a lung capacity of 5,800 mL and the average female's capacity is 4,300 mL.[78] We are plagued by the consistent underuse of our lungs.

This causes problems throughout the body, compounding physical and mental ailments. When we experience anxiety or panic, the heart races, the chest tightens, and the shoulders round as we gasp for air. This physical constriction further exacerbates the experience by restricting airflow as the heart races. Yogic science does not claim to replace modern medicine or to "fix" the complex dynamics within the human condition that aid in panic and anxiety. Yogic science does, however, teach you how to work with your physical form to manipulate your body into its most natural state of being. By intentionally bringing prana into your system during an anxiety or panic attack, you can create a chain reaction of self-healing responses.

Yoga is never a substitute for modern medicine, but it can aid in your body's ability to work with a regime more effectively. Think of it like taking a probiotic for your overall digestive health. Probiotics add living organisms to your gut biome that aid in the breakdown of nutrients. These organisms help nutrients assimilate, allowing your body to perform its natural functions more efficiently. Similarly, the pranayama techniques that manipulate the breath bring life-giving oxygen to the entirety of the lungs. The oxygenated blood pumped through the heart allows every other organ in the body to function more efficiently.

---

78. Frothingham, "What Is Expiratory Reserve Volume and How Is It Measured?"

Breathwork to Calm Anxiety
1. Breathe in for a count of four
2. Hold the breath for four
3. Exhale for a count of four
4. Hold the breath on the exhale for four
5. Repeat for one minute

Yogic science provides a foundational understanding of how to breathe correctly and why we do it. As you become intimately in tune with your body's functions, limitations, and expansive possibilities, you will find new ways to stretch and strengthen yourself. Pranayama is the expansion of your vital life force energy, your prana, throughout your body. This prana is used to awaken and balance the energy of the nadis and the chakras. The balancing of this energy is utilized to remove blockages within the body, providing clear energy channels for your Kundalini energy to flow unencumbered. This free-flowing energy ignites the nadi and chakras and eventually awakens the dormant Kundalini Shakti. The first step to removing any of your blockages is pranayama breathing techniques.

A Full Yogic Breath

To gain prana's maximum benefits, we first learn how to take a full yogic breath. Humans breathe every day, yet we take this fundamental operating process for granted. We can survive approximately three weeks without food and three days without water, but we can only survive a mere three minutes without air.[79] It is difficult to wrap our heads around how this is possible, especially because humans think about food and water far more often than they think about their breath. As mentioned previously, the majority of people are shallow breathers. We take short breaths, so when oxygen enters the body, it only fills up the top portion of the lungs. As we come to understand the full capacity of the lungs, we recognize shallow breaths as more of a gasp for air rather than the oxygenating, life-giving medicine the body craves.

---

79. Helmenstine, "How Long You Can Live Without Food, Water, or Sleep."

Continually taking shallow breaths is similar to always filling your car's gas tank a quarter of the way full. Sure, your car will run, but it will be unable to sustain long distances and you will need to stop to fill up the tank more often. The vehicle's parts and components will break down faster, strained from the extra wear and tear caused by continually running on a virtually empty tank. The same goes for the body. Shallow breaths keep you alive, but they are a far cry from giving your body the ample oxygen it requires. Factor in the stressors of modern-day life and the majority of us are running on empty, arriving at the gas station on fumes every day.

Unlike shallow breathing, inhaling and exhaling with a yogic breath allows you to maximize your full lung capacity. Let's begin by mindfully focusing on the prana, or life force energy, used to move air into the lungs, oxygenating the blood.

Pranayama[80]

There are three parts to a yoga breath: inhalation (*pooraka*), exhalation (*rechaka*), and retention (*kumbhaka*). Each of these steps is critical to move energy throughout the body. We'll discuss retention at the end of an exhalation and retention at the end of an inhalation as we move through the practice's more advanced exercises. First, let's focus on these three fundamental components, what they are, and how and why we perform them.

Inhalation

The first aspect of pranayama is inhalation. Inhalation occurs as we breathe deeply from the abdomen, filling the chest with air. The stomach expands from the body, filling the lungs and sending air up toward the throat. The difference in this yogic breath is that intention is focused on the spine's base and the belly's base to begin with. Like the analogy of filling up a cup, start at the bottom to maximize this life force energy. A critical aspect of the pranayama inhale is that you must intentionally allow the belly to extend and fill like an inflated ball, protruding in front of the body. The simple act of doing this can send forth a kaleidoscope of emotions and insecurities.

The protruding of the belly will feel awkward at first. We expand like a ball filled with air, not dissimilar to the uncomfortable feelings of bloating or gas. Instead of merely

---

80. *Prana* = Universal life force. *Yama* = Extension/expansion or control.

focusing on the belly moving outward, envision air filling up the abdomen, beginning first at the mooladhara and moving up the chakra system.

This action moves in three parts. First, the breath moves up from the belly's base, swelling the abdomen like a balloon. Next, the air pushes out of the ribs and chest as it expands. Finally, the upper chest and clavicle broaden as every nook and cranny of the torso is filled with prana's life force energy.

Pranayama Inhalation Process

1. Abdomen: Fill the abdomen or belly with air
2. Chest: Fill the rib cage and lungs with air
3. Clavicle: Fill the upper chest and collarbone area with air

Retention

In a full yogic breath, retention is performed at the top of the inhale. Retention is the pause between breaths. It is holding the breath in the moments that are neither an inhale nor an exhale. After you have pushed your physical body's limits to capacity, filled to the brim with air, you hold. The breath is controlled so that the oxygen brought within circulates throughout your system, filling every crevice of your extremities with this life force energy.

You will notice as you practice retention that pressure begins to build as you hold. Your body may start to shake as your throat tightens with oxygen begging to be released from your system. Later, when we discuss the concept of bandhas, you will learn how to harness this pressure through yogic locks to push past blockages and stagnation within the body. By practicing bandhas and full yogic breaths, we work to circulate this energy through the extremities, mind, heart, and soul.

When you withhold your breath, focus on the sensations felt as you deprive your body of the inhale or exhale. All manner of reactions will occur when you do this. It is not uncommon to begin yawning, fidgeting, thinking of seemingly unimportant things, or finding yourself overcome with a range of emotions. Retention after a long inhale circulates prana throughout the body's entirety. Retention after a long exhale forces the body to stay calm and "fight" for survival with an empty tank, as there is no oxygen in the system. Either of these extremes is bound to bring up emotions and resistance. Each is perfectly normal and part of the mental agility of the practice of yoga.

Natural Breathing

Contrary to a full yogic breath, retention is performed on both the inhale and exhale every time you breathe. Natural breathing consists of an inhale, a pause, an exhale, and a pause. The retention is short, virtually unrecognizable because you naturally breathe in this manner every day. You likely don't realize it, but you do hold your breath for a split second after each inhale and exhale. What sets yogic breathing apart is that it is the intentional holding of the breath for an extended amount of time with a purpose and desired result in mind.

NATURAL BREATHING PROCESS
1. Inhalation
2. Retention
3. Exhalation
4. Retention

Exhalation

The third component of pranayama is exhalation. Exhalation occurs as you release the air from your body in the descending order from which it came. First from behind the clavicle, then the rib cage, and finally the stomach. A full exhale is completed with the abdomen completely emptied, belly button pressing back toward the spine. Just as emotions may have stirred as you watched your body extend with the inhale's inflation, so too may you experience emotional fatigue as you watch the body become concave on the exhale.

Practice Pranayama on an Empty Stomach

As you practice and your body's muscle memory becomes more accustomed to this technique, you will notice your abdomen extending further from your core and the belly becoming more concave on the exhale. Envision your belly button moving backward as if it could touch your spine; this is the act of emptying the stomach that is necessary to gain the full benefits of the pranayama techniques. When the body digests, it is experiencing one of the most energy-consuming functions. The ability to circulate prana effectively restricts, and the ability to expel or fill air completely is compromised.

Pranayama exercises help expel toxins from the body, but if the body is digesting food, you will have a challenging time executing the techniques effectively. Most of us have both seen and felt the intestinal cavities distend from overeating or gas. This presents as pain and discomfort as the abdomen stretches and the body fights to expel foreign components from its system. Your yoga practice is about working with your body, not against it. Therefore, if you perform powerful breathing techniques like Breath of Fire having just consumed a large meal, you will be immensely uncomfortable and incapable of executing the technique properly.

The Five Divisions of Prana

As we move forward in the practice of pranayama, let's take a deeper dive into pranic energy and where and how it is directed within the body. *Prana* is life force energy. The word *yama* means control, and *ayama* translates as extension or expansion.[81] When the definitions of these words are combined, we understand *pranayama* as the control of the extension or expansion of life force energy. Through the manipulation of breath, you control the course of your prana, directing it within your body.

Pancha Prana[82]

There are five divisions of prana:

1. Prana: Flows through the lungs, heart, and nostrils

2. Apana: Flows from the lower abdomen to the elimination organs

3. Samana: Flow of nutrition, which processes through the abdominal organs

4. Udana: Flows from the heart to the head to the brain

5. Vyana: Flows through the entire body, including all limbs

---

81. Satyananda Saraswati, *Asana Pranayama Mudra Bandha*, 369.

82. *Pancha* = Five. *Prana* = Universal life force.

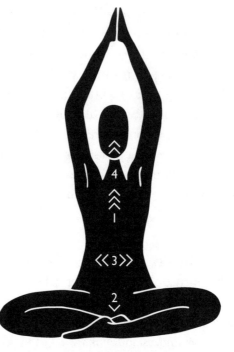

Pancha Prana

PRANA

Of the five divisions, the first is prana. This is the flow of energy that runs from the bottom of the lungs up through the chest cavity. Associated with heart and lung function, this energy flow is a forward or upward motion. As expressed in the yogic breath inhalation, this energy flows through the abdomen, chest cavity, clavicle, and out of the nose. This first division of air is what is traditionally thought of when envisioning prana, as it directly links to your breath.

APANA

Next is apana. This division of your prana focuses on the removal of fluids from the body. Visually represented from the belly button downward, this is the excretion of urine and other bodily excrements. As you breathe deeply, you work within the body's parameters to remove toxins and foreign bodies from your system. One of the many ways in which you do this is through the excretion of this energy. This occurs through the lower region of your system—the large intestine, kidneys, anus, and genitals.[83]

SAMANA

Third is samana, the retention, connecting your prana with your apana.[84] Samana resides in the abdomen, merging the upper and lower regions of this air/force. Its action is the moment when the body converts food to fuel. Food components are extracted in the digestive tract by way of the liver, intestines, pancreas, and stomach.[85] Samana helps you digest these nutrients, providing assimilation and distribution throughout the body, transforming this energy and preparing what does not serve you for removal. It is for this reason that the samana is considered the center for transformation.

UDANA

The fourth of the five vital forces is udana. Udana governs the head and the neck, moving energy upward from the throat to the face and senses. The location of the upa pranas, this region also manages the five minor pranas that work to expel energy from the body. The direction of its power up and out of this region stimulates the eyes, tongue, nose, and ears.[86] With its force activating these sensory hubs, this prana acts to provide the basis for overall awareness and consciousness, allowing you to interact effectively with the outside world.

VYANA

The fifth of the pancha pranas is vyana. Vyana is the entirety of the body, where all four of the other pancha pranas (prana, apana, samana, and udana) connect, creating collective energy throughout the body. Vyana ties together the prana divisions, reminding us that none of our functions are separate from one another. Each function impacts the collective with every action. Through pranayama practice, you intentionally direct this energy throughout your system, performing techniques to ignite and move the prana in

---

83. Satyananda Saraswati, *Asana Pranayama Mudra Bandha*, 371.

84. Victoria State Government Department of Health, "Digestive System Explained."

85. Satyananda Saraswati, *Asana Pranayama Mudra Bandha*, 372.

86. Satyananda Saraswati, *Asana Pranayama Mudra Bandha*, 372.

all five of these divisions. Here, you give your body the power it requires to move past blockages and expel all that no longer serves you rapidly and effectively.

Upa Pranas (Minor Pranas)

Upa pranas, or minor pranas, reside under the fourth of the five prana divisions, the udana. These actions are how the body cleans itself as a secondary activity, compared to the body's significant cleansing actions like intake, retention, and excretion.

NAGA

The act of burping as a medium for the body to cleanse itself may never have crossed your mind, yet according to yogic science, this is its primary function. Naga, or the act of burping, the first of the five upa pranas, allows you to remove unwanted air, gas, and toxins from the body. This minor prana forces unwanted air from the body.

KOORMA

The second of the upa pranas is koorma, or blinking. As you blink, you use the rapid motion of your eyelids to force air into this region. You can even remove an unwanted object from the vicinity; if you have had a gust of wind blow dirt or sand in your direction, you are familiar with the eyelids' rapid, involuntary fluttering. This quick motion causes your eyes to water, which removes whatever is in your eye that might be harmful. This also occurs when you experience extreme sadness, joy, or grief. As tears well up, your body attempts to remove the emotional energy from your body via two of the nine gates: your eyes.

KRIKARA

Krikara is the third of the upa pranas, our hunger or thirst. This prana cleanses the body of impurities by flushing toxins through the acts of eating and drinking. Fiber-rich foods aid the system in moving unwanted waste from the body. Fluids, particularly water, aid in flushing toxins from the cells. This is why it is immensely important to drink copious amounts of water after getting a massage, for example. The pressure of bodywork releases fluids and toxins into the body that were previously encapsulated in the constrictions that caused physical pain. The water you ingest directly after a massage is much like running water used to clean your dishes; the pressure and volume pushes unwanted particles from your system and down the proverbial drain of your body, much like the drain in your kitchen sink. This removal of fluids is initiated by apana, the division of your prana from the belly button downward.

DEVADATTA

The fourth of the upa pranas is devadatta, the act of sneezing. As you sneeze, you remove unwanted particles and foreign bodies from the nose and sinuses. The act of sneezing during allergy season is a perfect illustration of this minor prana. When you are allergic to something—for example, pollen or pet dander—the entry of these agents into your body through the nose causes you to sneeze. Suppose these allergens make their way into your sinus cavities without being expelled from the body via devadatta. In that case, the irritants result in sinus headaches and painful pressure. The exercises that follow are an excellent way to relieve this tension. By actively forcing air into the sinuses, you remove impurities that shallow breathing and devadatta cannot.

DHANANJAYA

The fifth of the minor pranas occurs in the form of rigor mortis, or dhananjaya. This action occurs when you leave your human vessel in the action of death. Your body's last act of cleansing, dhananjaya removes all that does not serve you from this earthly plane.

The Inhale and Exhale of Pranayama

Let's take a moment to discuss the directionality of an inhale and exhale. When you lengthen the body—growing taller, longer, and in an upward motion—you take a long, deep inhale. As you take a moment to breathe deeply, notice the crown of the head rise toward the sky as your lungs fill with air and your rib cage expands. The same motion occurs when you take a long deep inhale in the morning and stretch your body awake, your toes actively pointing away from the body and your arms outstretched high above your head. On the inhale, you make room. You expand, allowing air to fill your lungs and oxygenated blood to pump through your body.

On the exhale, your body will naturally contract, allowing air and toxins to leave the lungs. In many of the instructions within this book, an exhale brings the belly button deep into the spine. As you perform a deep exhale, allow all air to empty from the body, noticing as the stomach contracts and forms a concave C. Not dissimilar to the movement known as a C-curve in Pilates, when air releases from the body, you pull your navel toward your spine, engaging the muscles of the abdomen. Imagine how your body would react if you were punched in the stomach. This blunt trauma would force you to exhale automatically. The phrase "getting the wind knocked out of you" is commonplace in modern vernacular. Sudden force to the abdomen puts pressure on the solar plexus. This pressure causes temporary paralysis to the diaphragm, making it difficult to breathe. I don't suggest intentionally causing trauma to your abdomen, but when you are in the throes of your practice, let this visualization be a reminder of your body's natural inclination to breathe out as the body folds into itself.

With the visualization of air leaving the abdomen in the forefront of your mind, impart the same train of thought to the act of twisting. As you ring out your torso during a twist, so too are you removing all the air from this region, detoxifying your body. You twist from the center of your torso on the exhale, filling your lungs and abdomen with air on the inhale.

When you perform side-bending movements, so too do you exhale. Much like the act of bringing the belly button to the spine, as an example, when you bend to the right, the right side body's surface area gets smaller. This portion of the body constricts, forcing air outward. As the body moves back to center, the crown of the head reaches toward the ceiling. As the body lengthens, air fills the lungs with life-giving pranic energy. Whenever you lengthen and create room for air to enter, you inhale. Whenever you constrict, reducing the space for this prana to reside within your body, you exhale.

The exercises of pranayama help you detoxify the body and aid in the ease of all other movements throughout your life. When lifting heavy objects, there is a reason why you take a large inhale before thrusting the weight into the air. You need the added oomph, the energy of prana, to hoist the weight into motion. When air fills your lungs, it also enters your blood and muscles, aiding in your body's ability to perform these feats of strength. You stand taller with the body oxygenated from life-giving prana, your spine lengthened with the expansion of the inhale. The breath lubricates the body, creating more room for the joints to move freely.

Pranic Energy

Tapas refers to the intensity with which you perform your spiritual practices. The activities classified as tapas range from fasting to pranayama. In the yogic tradition, pranayama, traditionally written *pranayama pramtapah*, is described as the greatest tapa.[87] The intense manner in which you perform pranayama exercises has heating, healing, and detoxifying results. If this is your first introduction to pranayama, the methods may come across as vigorous and intense. For example, the technique Breath of Fire builds heat within the body, burning off impurities and stoking your digestive fire. It is difficult to perform for even one minute at first, so you should take each technique in short increments and begin to acclimate to this new breathing method, slowly increasing the vigor and intensity over time.

As you begin pranayama exercises, remember the lessons learned in the chapters prior. If you have tight shoulders, you will not be able to breathe effectively into the lungs. Do not discount each exercise's emotional component; pay close attention to how the practices make you feel. Do you have an easier time inhaling deeply or exhaling the air completely out of your lungs? What about retention? Does holding your breath send you into a fight-or-flight response? Do you feel uncomfortable while performing Bahir Kumbhaka, the mindful retention of the breath after exhalation? From a place of curiosity and exploration, pay attention to your physiological responses to each pranayama phase, but don't judge your response.

With each exhalation, you experience a death, and with each inhalation, an act of rebirth. Pay close attention to the visceral reaction you have to the words *death* and *rebirth*. Begin working with your pranayama practice by acknowledging the emotional response you have at the mere mention of this life cycle. Without judgment, can you begin to see the idea of death and rebirth from a place of beauty?

To move progressively forward, release the preconceived notions of the morbidity of these words via the knowledge gained from Kundalini's teachings. Acknowledge that each of the definitions behind pranayama's phases emphasizes mindful inhalation, exhalation, and retention of the breath. Each action is performed with intent and accuracy to elicit the desired result—the death of what no longer serves you and the birth of what does. Focus on these words and their meaning to remove the charge they have over your heart, mind, body, and soul. By merely acknowledging their potential to trigger, you begin releasing the energetic blockages wreaking havoc within your system, even before the first exercise is performed.

---

87. Ishwardas Chunilal Yogic Health Center, *Prayer and Mantrajapa*, 9.

Aspects of Pranayama
1. Pooraka (Shwasa): Inhalation

2. Rechaka (Prashwasa): Exhalation

3. Kumbhaka: Retention

4. Bahir Kumbhaka: External retention; mindful retention after exhalation

5. Aantir Kumbhaka: Internal retention; mindful retention after inhalation[88]

With each technique, you train the mind to observe as well as purify. The benefits of your pranayama practice, which compound with each repetition, help you further clarify the mind. Sweeping away your mind's cobwebs allows you to see, think, and feel more clearly because the effectiveness of these techniques removes blockages and aligns the body's hemispheres. With the blockages removed, energy flows evenly through both the ida and the pingala, allowing you to gain and maintain your footing through the ups and downs of life. As your prana moves freely up the sushumna, paving the way for Kundalini energy to rise, you gain access to the wisdom of your highest self. The wisdom that was inherent and available to you all along is now made accessible due to the ancient yogic science techniques that follow.

Exercises: Breathe Like a Yogi

These are nine pranayamas that often make up the foundation of a Kundalini practice:

1. Chandra Bhedana (Left Nostril Breathing)

2. Surya Bhedana (Right Nostril Breathing)

3. Nadi Shodhana (Alternate Nostril Breathing)

4. Kapalabhati (Skull Shining Breath)

5. Ujjayi (Ocean Breath)

6. Sheetali (Hissing Breath)

7. Sheetkari (Hissing Breath Variation)

8. Bhastrika (Bellows Breath or Breath of Fire)

9. Brahmari (Bee Breath)

---

88. Satyananda Saraswati, *Asana Pranayama Mudra Bandha*, 370.

This section will introduce pranayamas four, five, six, seven, and nine. Pranayamas one through three were covered in the exercise section of chapter 4, and the eighth pranayama was introduced in chapter 1.

The wisdom of the pranayamas provides life-altering pranic energy to you regardless of how far you roam. Try each one. Practice until you feel comfortable moving your breath with intention, mindfully observing and taking note of each ebb and flow. As you begin to feel more comfortable, make each practice your own, focusing your attention on the handful of practices that alleviate agitations and stressors. These techniques are always available to you, wherever and whenever you might need them.

✒ *Technique* ✑
Kapalabhati Pranayama (Skull Shining Breath)[89]

Cautions: Avoid if pregnant or suffering from high blood pressure.

Duration: One minute.

Posture: Sit comfortably in an easy pose with a straight spine, eyes forward and palms resting gently on the knees.

Technique: With the lips sealed, forcefully exhale from the nose, bringing the belly button to the spine.

Action: To begin, inhale through the nose with a straight spine, completing a full yogic breath. A full exhalation empties the abdomen, bringing the belly button to the spine. Perform another deep inhalation, followed by another full exhalation. Begin repetitive forceful exhalations, focusing on pressing the belly button deep into the spine. The inhalation will come naturally. Upon completion, with eyes closed, the hands rest on the knees as you allow the breath to return to natural breathing.

Repetition: Repeat forceful exhalations for one minute. Then meditate.

Checking the Technique: Bring the pointer, middle, and ring fingers of the right hand directly below the belly button. Begin kapalabhati breathing. Feel these three fingers moving in toward the body with each exhale. If your knees, shoulders, head, spine, or hips are also moving, draw the attention back to these three fingers. You are focusing

---

89. *Kapal* = Skull. *Bhati* = Shining.

on only this area. Repeat the technique with the fingers on the abdomen as the rest of the body remains still during practice.

This practice is similar to the Breath of Fire introduced in chapter 1, but it differs in the rhythmic way that the breath moves in and out. Breath of Fire is forceful, focusing on rapidly removing all of the air from the body in quick motions. This technique is a forceful exhale with a natural inhale. The difference can be found in the cadence; for every kapalabhati breath, you will have performed two to four Breaths of Fire.

Benefits: Can improve digestion, which increases appetite, and aids in the detoxification of the body.

∽ Technique ∽
Ujjayi Pranayama (Ocean Breath)[90]

Cautions: Avoid if suffering from hyperthyroidism.

Duration: One minute.

Posture: Sit comfortably in an easy pose with a straight spine, the eyes forward and palms resting gently on the knees.

Technique: Ujjayi contracts the glottis, the space between the two vocal cords, while inhaling and exhaling through the nose.

Action: To begin, inhale through the nose with a straight spine, filling the body with air from the spine's base. A full exhalation empties the abdomen, again through the nose, as you bring the belly button to the spine. On the next inhalation, restrict the glottis as the lips remain sealed, creating a vibration in the throat. On the following exhalation, a more resonant vibration occurs as the air passes over the restricted glottis. Repeat inhalation and exhalation. Upon completing all reps, allow the breath to return to natural breathing, eyes closed and hands resting on the knees.

Repetition: Repeat inhalation and exhalation for one minute. Then meditate.

Checking the Technique: Envision air filling up the body from the spine's base, vibrating in the throat as it passes the constricted glottis. On the exhale, visualize fogging up a mirror as the mouth remains closed and all air leaves the body.

---

90. *Ut* = Up. *Jjayi* = Go.

Benefits: Can open the upper chakras (heart, throat, third eye, and crown). Aids in the reduction of high blood pressure and improves vocal cord strength.

✎ *Technique* ✐
Sheetali Pranayama (Hissing Breath)

Cautions: Avoid if suffering from low blood pressure, a cold, excess mucus, or sinusitis.

Duration: One minute.

Posture: Sit comfortably in an easy pose with a straight spine, eyes forward and palms resting gently on the knees.

Technique: With the mouth slightly open, roll the tongue into a U shape as the lips gently close around the tongue.

Action: Soften the eyes to close, focusing your internal gaze on the third eye. Begin inhaling through the opening in the tongue, filling the body with air. Exhale air back out through the tongue. Repeat the inhalation and exhalation. Upon completing all reps, allow the breath to return to natural breathing, eyes closed and hands resting on the knees.

Repetition: Repeat inhalation and exhalation for one minute. Then meditate.

Checking the Technique: Envision air entering the mouth through the rolled tongue, filling and cooling the body. Air exits the body the same way it entered, passing through the rolled tongue on its way out of the mouth.

Benefits: Can aid in appetite control, facilitates the reduction of hyperacidity, and allows for relaxation while maintaining alertness. Cools body temperature, which can lead to reduction of fever.

✎ *Technique* ✐
Sheetkari Pranayama (Hissing Breath Variation)

Cautions: Avoid if suffering from low blood pressure, a cold, excess mucus, or sinusitis.

Duration: One minute.

Posture: Sit comfortably in an easy pose with a straight spine, eyes forward and palms resting gently on the knees.

Technique: The mouth is closed, lips gently pressing against one another, the upper and lower teeth together. The tip of the tongue presses against the back of the teeth.

Action: Gently bring the eyes to close, focusing your internal gaze on the third eye. Begin inhaling through the teeth, filling the body with air. Exhale air back out through the teeth. Repeat the inhalation and exhalation. Upon completing reps, allow the breath to return to natural breathing, eyes closed and hands resting on the knees.

Repetition: Repeat inhalation and exhalation for one minute. Then meditate.

Checking the Technique: Envision the air entering the mouth through the teeth, creating a C sound as it enters the body. Then envision air exiting the body the same way it entered, passing through the teeth and out of the mouth. Sheetkari pranayama is utilized by those who cannot roll their tongue.

Benefits: Can aid in appetite control, facilitates the reduction of hyperacidity, and cools body temperature.

∼ *Technique* ∼
Bhramari Pranayama (Bee Breath)

Cautions: Avoid if suffering from an ear infection.

Duration: One minute.

Posture: Sit comfortably in an easy pose with a straight spine, eyes forward and palms resting gently on the knees.

Technique: Bhramari creates the sound of a bee as you exhale through the nose. The mouth is closed, lips gently pressing against one another, the upper and lower teeth together. The tip of the tongue presses against the back of the teeth with the inhalation and exhalation occurring through the nose.

Action: Inhale through the nose and, with a straight spine, fill the body with air from the spine's base. A full exhalation empties the abdomen, again through the nose, bringing the belly button to the spine. Deeply inhale. On the exhalation, begin creating the sound of a bee by humming with the lips remaining closed. Inhale without sound, then make the humming bee sound with each exhalation. Upon completing all reps, allow the breath to return to natural breathing, eyes closed and hands resting on the knees.

Repetition: Repeat inhalation and exhalation for one minute. Then meditate.

Checking the Technique: With the lips closed, feel the vibration of the breath on the lips, inside the mouth, and rising into the sinuses. Visualize the wave rising behind the eyes, engulfing the third eye and the crown chakras. Bhramari creates the external sound of a bee as one exhales through the nose.

Benefits: May strengthen the nervous system, improve creativity, and reduce the symptoms of sinusitis. Can aid in the alleviation of writer's block and provide a reduction in negative self-talk.

Eight
Gesture Like a Yogi
(Directing Energy with Mudras)

In this chapter, we tap into the vibration of the planets and elements through the subtle yet powerful energy residing in the fingertips. Mudras are gestures—the most common mudras in our Kundalini practice are the ones made with the hands. We use mudras to manipulate energy and communicate intent. As we move forward on our yoga journey, how can we bring more intentionality to all we do, including talking with our hands?

What Is a Mudra?

A mudra is a gesture or attitude. Gestures refer to the action of your movements or positions. In contrast, an attitude refers to a much more esoteric byproduct of these actions. Now that you are deep into your Kundalini journey, you are becoming aware of the practice's subtle emotional, mental, and physical effects. Mudras are a perfect example of a small thing having a profound impact. These mental faculties are described as psychic, emotional, and devotional.[91] The attitudes of energy flow link your prana with the greater collective's strength.

Mudra stems from the Sanskrit word *mud*, meaning delight or pleasure, and *dravay*, or *dru*, meaning to draw forth. Commonly defined as a shortcut or circuit bypass,

---

91. Satyananda Saraswati, *Asana Pranayama Mudra Bandha*, 421.

mudras are used to redirect the flow of energy within the body.[92] These gestures are subtle, not nearly as strong as the pipe-unclogging energy created with bandhas, but powerful nonetheless. Mudras redirect your power to improve your concentration and awareness. People regularly fall prey to the monkey mind, tapping into the continuous running loop of scattered internal dialogue. The use of mudras, particularly in a meditative state, helps calm this chaos. Like redirecting your attention with your drishti, mudras give your brain the gentle redirection it needs to come back to center.

Mudras are deemed so influential and essential that they are considered a science of their own in many of the ancient texts. The attention needed to practice mudras effectively is noted as the attention of higher consciousness. This is one of the many reasons mudras are being introduced in chapter 8 instead of at the beginning of the book. With the foundations of Kundalini in place, you have gained a level of reflective awareness that will allow you to tap into the gesture's subtle nuances; you are now capable of harnessing their magic.

The Types of Mudras

When envisioning mudras, you most likely envision the hand gestures used during a yoga class. Gyan Mudra, the most well-known mudra, is the act of bringing the tip of the pointer finger to the thumb. This is an attitude you might have executed while sitting for meditation or outstretched in a dancer pose. But mudras are more than a simple hand gesture. Mudras fall into five distinct categories: hand mudras, head mudras, postural mudras, lock mudras, and perineal mudras.

Hasa, or hand mudras, are the most commonly used, such as the Gyan Mudra. *Mana*, or head mudras, are commonly executed during yoga classes, though why they are classified as mudras or the reasoning behind these techniques is not known. *Kaya* are postural mudras also performed in a standard sequence of most yoga. *Bandha*, or lock mudras, are paramount to Kundalini's practice. Lastly, *adhara* are perineal mudras. This is a potent mudra that utilizes the sex organs to achieve desired results.

We will first discuss the four lesser-known types of mudras, again providing a solid foundation of knowledge to build on. You may not use all five mudra types in your Kundalini practice, but with this grounding knowledge in place, you will begin to cultivate the healing energy of mudras more effectively. Knowledge is power, and the more

---

92. Satyananda Saraswati, *Asana Pranayama Mudra Bandha*, 421.

you learn about mudras, the greater your potential to harness their power to cultivate your most aligned life.

Mana (Head Mudras)

A head mudra utilizes the eyes, ears, nose, tongue, or lips intentionally. As an example, in Shambhavi Mudra the gaze focuses at the center of the eyebrows. Commonly referred to as "eyebrow center gazing," this drishti is a foundational technique for one's meditation practice. Holding the gaze, releasing the focus, holding, and releasing again allows the eyes to close, the mind to soften, and the meditation to begin.

An example of a technique utilizing the tongue is Khechari Mudra, or tongue lock. This mudra is subtle, but its connection to the tongue and the salivary glands cultivates the ability for one to overcome hunger and thirst. The nuance of these simple techniques is working on such an innate level that people often don't immediately recognize the benefits. You will understand the change later down the line when you look back, observing the shift.

It is suggested to perform head mudras for three to five minutes during the beginner stage. This allows you to gain control over the posture and to gain confidence about executing the mudra correctly. As this baseline is established, start to add these gestures to the more complex kriyas. Should you perform a kriya where you feel off or unable to match the technique's cadence, take a moment to break down the individual components, resolidifying your execution of the basics. Mana mudras are a perfect place to start. By looking at the head positions in greater detail and taking three minutes to practice with pinpointed attention, you re-ground yourself.

Regaining control over the moment is another excellent example of how mudras can aid us in everyday life. When you feel overwhelmed, pause and bring it back to basics. One minute of slow, intentional gazing at the tip of the nose can refocus your thoughts, helping you process situations from a calm and levelheaded state of mind before proceeding.

Bandha (Lock Mudras)

Mudra bandhas, or lock mudras, are executed in tandem with the implementation of bandhas. You will learn about bandhas in the next chapter; therefore, we will not go into the depths of their magic here, but what we will do is touch briefly on these three locks. The lock mudras are Maha Mudra, Maha Bheda Mudra, and Maha Vedha Mudra. These mudras combine with prana to prepare one's body for a Kundalini awakening.[93]

---

93. Satyananda Saraswati, *Asana Pranayama Mudra Bandha*, 421.

The Maha Mudra links the energy of the ajna and mooladahara chakras. As discussed in previous chapters, when these two chakras are activated—first the ajna, then the mooladhara—a continual energy loop charges with prana, aiding in the removal of energetic blocks.[94] Maha Bheda Mudra is said to supercharge the mind-body connection, while Maha Vedha Mudra is a powerful mudra for turning inward and enhancing one's extrasensory gifts.[95] Each of these mudras are intrinsic, working on a deep and, at the same time, highly spiritual and interconnected level.

We will go into more detail in chapter 9, but bandhas are to be explored slowly and with heightened awareness. Take care to monitor the physical and emotional ripple effect these powerful mudras have.

Kaya (Postural Mudras)

Unlike a kriya, or asana flow, kayas typically utilize only one position to invoke one's psychic awareness. The word *psychic* might be jarring or off-putting to some, therefore we first focus on reframing this translation.

Psychic awareness can be replaced by the phrases *extrasensory gifts* or *heightened intuition*. These terms are seamlessly interchangeable, but the word *psychic* does not need to be shied away from. It is through increased Kundalini practice that you are able to hear the voice of your intuition more clearly, and you will be better at picking up on the nonverbal cues of others. This can increase your empathy as well as provide a clear path for your own self-compassion. Because these postural mudras increase the intuitive awareness of the practitioner, the most commonly used techniques have the term *psychic* in the translation.

Viparita Karani Mudra translates to "an inverted psychic attitude." This posture, similar to the shoulder stand, adds ujjayi pranayama and concentrates on the manipura and vishuddhi chakras. This inversion works to recirculate the blood, awaken the body, increase the metabolism, and tone the stomach muscles. The second most widely used technique is Pashinee Mudra, the folded psychic attitude. In this mudra, the opposite approach is taken. Unlike the lengthening of the body in Viparita Karani Mudra's inversion, in Pashinee Mudra, you fold forward into yourself, with the knees, shins, ankles, feet, shoulders, neck, and head on the ground. Awareness is evoked as the focus turns to

---

94. Satyananda Saraswati, *Asana Pranayama Mudra Bandha*, 461.

95. Satyananda Saraswati, *Asana Pranayama Mudra Bandha*, 463–65.

the mooladhara and vishuddhi chakras with long, slow, rhythmic breathing. This psychic mudra balances the nervous system because the sensory deprivation slows the breath and the mind's rhythm while stimulating the spinal nerves and abdominal organs.

These physical mudras are much more than the postures or asanas of a standard yoga class. These mudras (and all mudras) focus heavily on the mental concentration of the positions. For example, the pose of Viparita Karani Mudra is very similar to a shoulder stand, but the goal is not merely to invert the body and work the abdominal muscles. Once you are thoroughly versed in Kundalini, you work to tap into your spiritual side with each technique. You begin to feel the subterranean shifts occurring with each "sit."

Adhara (Perineal Mudras)

The next category of mudras is the adhara, or perineal mudras. As these mudras are noted to engage sexual energy, they can easily be misunderstood or used in a way that does not honor the intention behind the techniques.

Perineal mudras redistribute your sexual energy, moving it upward through your body to the brain.[96] Your sexual energy is one of creation; it does not merely refer to the act of sex or procreation. Use the energy created by these mudras to birth new ideas, friendships, work opportunities, and ways of being. This energy center allows you to tap into your femininity in ways that create ease and joy in your life. Just as the term *psychic* may be triggering to some, the phrase *sexual energy* may also cause discomfort. As you perform these techniques, I encourage you to think of your sexual energy as your creativity and your ability to birth a new, more whole, more aligned version of yourself.

There are only two mudras in this category: Ashwini Mudra and Vajroli/Sahajoli Mudra. Ashwini Mudra, more commonly referred to as horse gesture, engages the rapid contraction and relaxation of the anus. The second mudra varies slightly based on if you were born with male or female genitalia. Vajroli Mudra, the posture for those with male genitalia, and Sahajoli Mudra, the pose for those with female genitalia, work with the sexual organs. Both exercises increase the strength of your pelvic floor and the muscles surrounding each of the lower gates. In yogic science, gates refer to the openings of the body, such as that of the ears, nose, and mouth. The two lower gates refer to the openings of the body found in our lower antomy used to remove fluid and waste from the body.

---

96. Satyananda Saraswati, *Asana Pranayama Mudra Bandha*, 424.

Hasta (Hand Mudras)

The most widely used mudras in Kundalini practice are hastas, or hand mudras. The bulk of the mudras utilized in Kundalini are meditative. Just like all mudras, these hand positions redirect the flow of pranic energy back within the body. Similar to closing an energy loop or the fluid motion of an infinity symbol, when you connect your fingertips together, you redirect, move, and bend your energy internally in a continuous loop.

In chapter 6, we discussed the importance of the leg position to close the loop of energy at the body's base, redirecting the energy inward instead of downward. The bending of the knees and feet redirects the prana up from the extremities into the trunk, igniting the chakras and recirculating this flow. With that knowledge and its implementation in the techniques prior, you now learn the importance of also engaging the hands while in these positions.

Both the soles of the feet and the palms of the hands are receptors. We receive and expel energy from both of these locations, just as we do from the crown of the head. When you are cold, one of the quickest ways to bring warmth into your body is to place socks on your feet, gloves on your hands, and a hat on your head. This is similar to the image of practicing Kundalini with the feet turned in, the fingertips in a mudra, and a turban on the head. So too does Kundalini warm and engage the body by directing its natural healing abilities inward.

Gyan Mudra

The most commonly used mudra is Gyan Mudra. This is when you connect the pointer finger and thumb. The execution of this is seen most frequently with the palms facing up and the back of the hand and wrist resting on the knees. *Gyan* means knowledge or wisdom. By connecting these two fingers in this manner, you are working to activate the knowledge within. Through this gesture, you are tapping into the infinite knowledge and wisdom of the Universe.

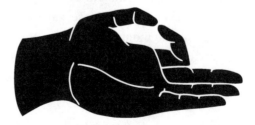

Gyan Mudra

BHAIRAVA MUDRA

In Bhairava Mudra, sometimes called Buddha Mudra, you rest your right hand in your left with the palms facing up. This gesture is most often used when sitting in an easy pose. The back of the left hand rests in your lap.

When the left hand is placed on top of the right, the mudra has changed to Bhairavi Mudra. The left hand represents the feminine, so Bhairavi Mudra is considered the female counterpart of Bhairava Mudra.[97]

With either hand position on top, this mudra represents the connection of the ida and the pingala, the masculine and feminine nadis, to the divine.

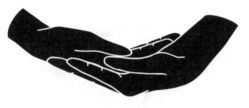

Bhairava Mudra

DHYANA MUDRA

Another variation of Bhairava Mudra is Dhyana Mudra. In this gesture, the right hand rests in the palm of the left at the navel. Bring the thumbs together to touch. The connected thumbs form a soft triangle in the negative space as they turn up toward the sky. This mudra is often referred to as the mudra of enlightenment, helping you hone your concentration and gain power over the mind.

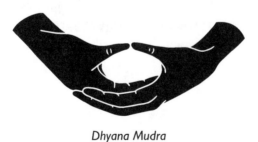

Dhyana Mudra

---

97. Satyananda Saraswati, *Asana Pranayama Mudra Bandha*, 429.

YONI MUDRA

Another commonly used mudra is the Yoni Mudra. *Yoni* refers to a woman's womb. As we are each born from a womb, invoking this womb energy is similar to connecting with Source. Source refers to the place from where we all come. Other names for Source are God, the Infinite, the Universe, and the Eternal Mother. All descriptions are interchangeably used to explain the "source" of this connection.

This gesture's shape outlines the same shape as a woman's womb, positioned in front of the body at the same height and elevation.[98] Make this gesture to expand into creation, creating new opportunities, emotions, desires, and beginnings in your life.

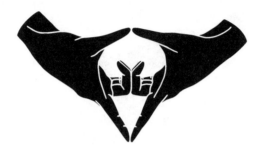

Yoni Mudra

ANJALI MUDRA

Lastly, we discuss the most universal of all hand mudras, Anjali Mudra, sometimes called Prayer Pose. The symbol of prayer, Anjali Mudra, is used across most demographics and faiths. *Anjali* means to offer or salute, and *mudra* means to seal. Utilize this mudra to offer up and seal your practice. This is the reason Anjali Mudra is used at the end of a practice: You are closing the experience in an expression of gratitude, offering up all that you have done to your highest self and for the highest and best of all.

---

98. Satyananda Saraswati, *Asana Pranayama Mudra Bandha*, 427.

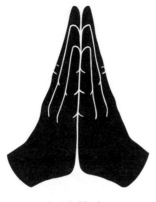

Anjali Mudra

Grounding and Receiving with Mudras

In moments when you feel anxious or overwhelmed, one of the quickest ways to re-center is to ground yourself. Through grounding, you reconnect to the earth. I find that the most effective way to bring myself back to center is to walk barefoot outdoors. The ability to live in a place where I may place my feet in the grass or sand is so paramount to my overall health that it now plays a crucial role in any decision-making process regarding my home and travel.

Reconnecting with the earth is the actual skin-to-element contact that occurs when you remove your shoes from the equation. Walking barefoot allows the earth's energy to soak up into the soles of your feet, which is an entry point that can bring this supportive, life-giving energy into your body. This action also allows what no longer serves you to escape through the pads of your feet, flowing into and transmuting within the earth.

If you can connect the soles of your feet directly to the earth, you are capable of calming your mind, recalibrating your body, and feeling the strength and support of Mother Earth within you. Even without this luxury, you can still tap into your mudra process to gain such freedom. By placing the palms down on your knees as you meditate, you mimic the soles of your feet connecting with the earth. As your palms face down toward the earth, the act of reconnecting to your limbs has a way of pushing you closer to this stabilizing energy. Bonus points for skin-to-skin contact, for just as with the connection of your bare feet to the land, feeling the skin of your body is another way of bringing yourself back home.

If you flip the palms up so that the backs of the hands rest on the knees, this results in an energetic intention to receive. Should you seek spiritual guidance, turning the palms upward may enhance your ability to speak to your guides, ancestors, angels, deities, spirit guides, and highest self. This creates an open channel to communicate with the divine. You are always divinely held, and through the act of surrender that accompanies this receiving mudra, you call forth your intuition and your highest self's knowledge.

Mudras, the Elements, and the Planets

In the spirit of grounding and the connection to Mother Earth, we will now discuss the connection between specific mudras and the elements. When studying the lineages of yoga, the intertwining of the foundations of Ayurveda is ever-present. The ancient science of Ayurveda uses food as medicine to heal the body and prevent disease.

Like yoga, Ayurveda addresses the five elements within each of our bodies: We nourish ourselves with food from the earth; we exist within the ether; we breathe air into the lungs; we stoke the digestive fire within when we eat; and we hydrate our bodies with the flow of water. Each element interacts with the body, providing necessary biological functions so we can thrive and exist on this earthly plane. The body works in harmony with the natural world.

Mudras Correspondences

Each finger corresponds to an element, a planet, and a specific energy.

THUMB
Element: Earth
Planet: Mars
Energy: Ego

You will notice that most mudras connect the thumb to another finger. Thumbs represent the earth. This is a grounding element that allows you to regain your footing and come home to yourself. Thumbs also represent your ego. Ego, in today's modern world, gets a bit of a bad rap. Deriving from the word *egotistical,* which is when you are overly focused on yourself, it's no wonder people have an aversion to the word. Many teachings speak of stripping oneself of the ego, the battle against the ego, or detaching from its energy altogether. The thought process surrounding ego is much different in Kundalini. Kundalini focuses on how to harness your ego for advancement and alignment instead of stripping the body of the ego or ignoring its existence altogether.

The thumb and ego are also connected to the planet Mars. Mars is the planet of war, and it's very common for people to feel at war with themselves, especially when fighting to balance internal darkness with the light. Kundalini teaches the importance of balancing both light and dark, masculine and feminine. Dipping back into these teachings and honing in on duality, you can now see that the ego, which is touted as the darkness, also has a side of it that can be considered light.

Ego is often reduced to an expression of self-centeredness, but consider its positive attributes. Have there been times when placing your best interest above others' was both necessary and for the highest and best of all? Could there be moments when you look at your ego as a superpower, tapping into your ability to uplift yourself, honor your needs, and make decisions from a place of high self-worth?

PINKY FINGER
Element: Water
Planet: Mercury
Energy: Friendship and prosperity

The pinky finger is associated with the planet Mercury. The pinky's connection to the thumb in Buddhi Mudra is said to connect the energy of friendship and prosperity.[99] Also associated with the water element, harnessing this element's power allows you to flow seamlessly through all discussions or negotiations. If you wish to overcome discord in a friendship or are struggling to place your interests over that of a friend or colleague, connect the pinky and thumb as you talk it out. You may witness the discord dissipate and notice the dialogue turn into a productive environment for all parties. Because it is also considered the link to prosperity, connecting your pinky finger to your thumb will help you overcome self-limiting beliefs or a lack of confidence.

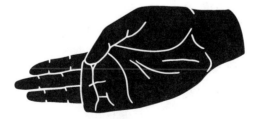

Buddhi Mudra

---

99. Singh Sahib, *Success and the Spirit*, 185.

Ring Finger
Element: Fire
Planets: Sun and Venus
Energy: Health

When discussing the sun, we begin by acknowledging that modern science has determined that the sun is not a planet, but as discussed throughout this book, the teachings of yogic science are based on the ancient Vedic texts. In these texts, the sun is an important part of the solar system, just as it is an immensely important part of the science of astrology. When these teachings originated, the sun was believed to be a planet, and for that reason it is noted here as such. The technical classification of this energy source is not as important here, for the teaching focuses on the energy this solar entity invokes and not the nomenclature it resides under.

As you bring the ring finger and thumb to touch, you create Surya Mudra. This sun line brings health.[100] The fire element is associated with the ring finger and the sun. The sun, which is a literal ball of flame, is connected to the belly and digestive ball of fire.

In astrology, the fire signs are Aries, Leo, and Sagittarius. Fire signs are associated with quick-wittedness and the ability to go, go, go. They will burn down anything standing in their way. The energy of fire signs embodies the element of fire and the strength of the sun. Fire signs have the ability to accomplish anything with a lively, fiery spirit or an overbearing, fiery temper. Depending on your perspective, you can see these energies as positive or negative. The challenge is to find grace on both ends of the spectrum. There are times when harnessing a vibrant spirit's energies may be just what the doctor ordered, and a fiery temper might save your life. See past the darkness and the light, choosing instead to live somewhere in the middle.

Another way of looking at the ring finger's connection to the thumb can be one of harnessing the energy of the sun. Yes, the sun is a fiery gas ball, but it is also an ever-present light of endurance. The sun is physically situated at the center of our universe. It is the sun that powers all life on earth. Without the sun, plants would not grow, the earth's bounty would freeze, and we would no longer survive as a human species.

Foster your connection to fire and the sun to harness the energy of true health of the mind, body, heart, and soul. The stamina of the sun helps you maintain this path. As

---

100. Singh Sahib, *Success and the Spirit*, 185.

we learned in chapter 5, digestive fire, representative of the sun, promotes health of the digestive system and helps the body assimilate life-sustaining nutrients.

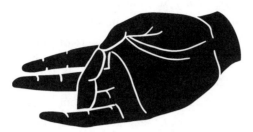

Surya Mudra

Middle Finger
Element: Air
Planet: Saturn
Energy: Purity and piety

Saturn, the element associated with the middle finger, brings forth wisdom and patience.[101] With Saturn's energy, we purify the mind, learning to allow things to transpire and unfold in divine timing. The irony of the middle finger being associated with wisdom, patience, and purity brings some levity to this practice. Returning to the discussion of light and dark, when the thumb is disconnected from the middle finger, it is the opposite of purity. Giving someone "the bird" or "flipping someone off" embodies this disconnection perfectly; this gesture lacks wisdom and patience with its hasty, emotionally charged action. It's an act of psychological projection.

Psychological projection is when you project undesired feelings or emotions onto someone else rather than dealing with undesirable feelings yourself. Ultimately, this is a defense mechanism. When you give someone the middle finger, you push all of your anger through the body and out the middle finger, directing it toward the person, place, or thing triggering that emotion. You may feel better in the moment because of the action's temporary release, but the seat of this emotional trigger still lies dormant within you.

Begin to disrupt this emotional projection pattern via your middle finger's connection to the thumb, also known as Shuni Mudra. The element of air represents the middle

---

101. Singh Sahib, *Success and the Spirit*, 185.

finger. This isn't a far leap when you envision the release of hot air that accompanies flipping someone the bird. Tap back into the earth element associated with the thumb. This connection might be a remedy for your temper.

Ayurveda teaches that the opposite of something is often the medicine. Sometimes these fits of passion and anger may feel like having an out-of-body experience. Grounding yourself with Shuni Mudra allows the energy to flow through you so that it may be transmuted and healed calmly. This simple gesture enables you to return to yourself before you fly off the handle. You can then tap into your intuition and get to the root of your emotion. The goal is to uncover the source of the trigger so that it no longer has control over you.

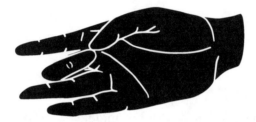

Shuni Mudra

POINTER FINGER
Element: Ether/space
Planet: Jupiter
Energy: Overcoming hurdles

The pointer fingers correlate to the planet Jupiter. The energy is that of overcoming hurdles and mastering expansion.[102] The element associated with the pointer or index finger is space, the expansive galaxy that encompasses all things within its existence. When we speak of space or the ether, we think of the Universe. In the world of spirituality, especially in the West, the Universe is terminology often interchanged with God or Source. This vastness encompasses all knowledge, guidance, and support available to us, divine or otherwise.

---

102. Singh Sahib, *Success and the Spirit*, 185.

By covering the thumb tightly in this mudra, you work to overcome the ego's hurdles. The mind passes what is believed to be relevant and correct, instead reaching toward what provides limitless expansion.

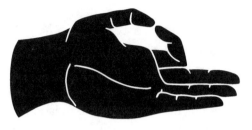

Gyan Mudra

As I progress on the path of Kundalini yoga, one of the most beautiful things I derive joy from is the interconnectedness of every religion, demographic, method of study, and modality. Through the simple study of connecting the thumb to one of your fingers, we touched on astrology, Ayurveda, religion, and language nuances. The more you grow as an individual and the more you seek out knowledge in the far corners of the globe, the more often these synchronicities come into focus. The phrase "same, but different" comes to mind. This phrase illustrates that we are all unique, yet we are all the same. The human race united as one, yet each of us beautifully diverse in our own idiosyncratic way.

The more you can look at the world from this lens, the quicker the interconnectedness comes into focus. Try harnessing the power of the pause cultivated within your yoga practice. More aha moments are brought to the forefront, as if the cumulation of every experience and teaching begins to move inward and combines at the core. Use these tools to intentionally draw on the energy of such synchronicities whenever possible. With simple hand mudras that can be executed virtually undetected in almost any situation, you have yet another tool in your tool belt, bringing you closer to your highest and best self, which has a ripple effect for the highest and best of all.

Connecting the Thumbs with Intention
- Connect the thumb to the index finger for wisdom.
- Connect the thumb to the middle finger to overcome challenges.

- Connect the thumb to the ring finger for energy and vitality.
- Connect the thumb to the pinky finger for a clear mind and improved communication.

Exercises: Gesture Like a Yogi

The following techniques focus on the subtle energies of mudras to create cosmic shifts with lasting results. When performing these techniques, focus your mind on the teachings of this chapter and the energy each meditation or gesture is intending to invoke. At this point in your Kundalini practice, you have a foundation from which you may now begin to incorporate the spiritual component of your practice. Where intention goes, energy flows. Focus your intention on your desired outcome as you proceed.

◠ *Technique* ◡
Excel, Excel, Fearless Meditation

Duration: Three minutes.

Posture: Sit in an easy pose, legs crossed, sit bones firmly on the ground with a straight spine.

Mudra: Adopt Gyan Mudra, resting the backs of the hands softly on the knees.

Drishti: The gaze focuses on the chin, with eyes 90 percent closed.

Mantra (Retention After Inhalation): "I am bountiful, I am blissful, I am beautiful."

Mantra (Retention After Exhalation): "Excel, excel, fearless."

Action: Deeply inhale. At the top of the inhale, internally chant the mantra, "I am bountiful, I am blissful, I am beautiful." Exhale deeply. At the bottom of the exhale, retain the breath and internally chant the mantra, "Excel, excel, fearless."

Repetition: Repeat the breathwork and mantras for three minutes.

Checking the Technique: As you rest Gyan Mudra on the knees, ensure the wrists are the main point of contact. The wrists' placement allows the spine, neck, and head to remain straight as the shoulders relax away from the ears and gently roll down the back.

Benefits: Can increase confidence and perseverance.

∽ *Technique* ∽
Guru Nanak's Treasure Meditation

Duration: Eleven minutes.

Posture: Sit comfortably in an easy pose with a straight spine.

Mudra: The right elbow bends as you bring the right hand, palm facing down, to the heart center. The left elbow bends to a right angle in alignment with the shoulder. The left bicep faces the ceiling. The triceps face down toward the earth. The left hand is in Gyan Mudra, palm facing forward.

Drishti: The eyes are 90 percent closed as the gaze focuses on the tip of your nose.

Mantra: "Har, har, har, har, haree, haree."

Cadence: Each "har" is one second long, and each "haree" stretches to two seconds.

Technique: The mantra is completed in one full exhale in a monotone voice.

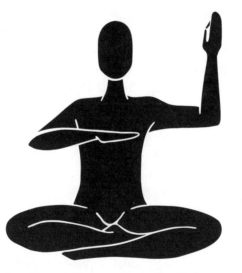

Guru Nanak's Treasure Meditation Technique

Action: The mudra remains the same throughout the kriya. As you take long inhales and exhales, monotonously chant the mantra.

Repetition: Repeat the mantra for eleven minutes. Meditate.

Checking the Technique: The left forearm is perpendicular to the ground, fingers pointing toward the sky. The left arm is held in an oath-taking position. The right arm is in front of the body aligned with the chest, palm facing down.

Benefits: Can build self-reliance and aids in increased productivity.

⌒ *Technique* ⌒
Meditation to Get Rid of "Couldn't"

Duration: Eleven minutes.

Posture: Sit comfortably in an easy pose with a straight spine.

Mudra: Cross your fingers, middle finger behind pointer finger. Bend the ring and pinky fingers, locking them in place using the thumbs. The elbows are bent so the mudra is at ear level.

Drishti: Eyes gently close as the internal gaze focuses on the third eye.

Mantra: Chant the mantra "har" from the navel.

Technique: With the arms bent (but not quite at a right angle), bring the mudra level with the ears and begin the mantra. The arms are in line with the body, not in front or behind. As you chant the mantra, bring the abdomen in toward the spine in a sharp jolt.

Action: This kriya's action is relatively simple. Maintain the same posture for the entirety of the meditation. The arms will most likely get tired because they are being held, without moving, for eleven minutes. If they do, drop them for a moment and then return to a meditative state.

Repetition: Repeat the mantra for eleven minutes. For the three final breaths, focus on the mantra and the energy created with this meditation. Allow it to circulate throughout the body. At the end of the third exhalation, release the hands, allowing the arms to rest on the knees. To close, inhale deeply, retaining the breath after the inhale to circulate the prana created with this technique. Repeat the three-part breath (inhalation, retention, and exhalation) three times. Meditate.

Checking the Technique: Your arms are engaged as you create the mudra. Take care not to strain in the upper body by relaxing the shoulders away from the ears and stretching and lengthening the neck. The muscles will fatigue and potentially begin shaking as strength builds. These reactions are normal, as you are pushing past mental and physical limitations. Attempt to maintain the posture for as long as possible. If your muscles fatigue, drop the arms and shake the hips, shoulders, torso, neck, arms, and head. After you release the tension in the entire body, situate yourself and begin again.

Benefits: Aids in the reduction of self-limiting beliefs. Can result in the mental strength to push through moments when you think you cannot do something.

Nine

Squeeze Like a Yogi (Push Past Blockages Using Bandhas)

WHAT POPS INTO YOUR mind when you hear the word *squeeze*? The pressing for the juice of a lemon, or maybe the tight embrace of a loved one? Squeezing is something we think little of when exercising, yet it is an action performed with each flex, squat, and twist. A yoga practice is filled with cues that instruct you to tighten throughout the body. The majority of the muscles you envision squeezing are the ones commonly known. Though it is crucial to work the larger muscle groups such as the biceps, triceps, quadriceps, and hamstrings, what about the smaller, intrinsic muscles that aid in your frame's function and stability? Through yoga, we take special care to focus our attention on the internal powerhouses that get little attention in mainstream fitness. This chapter is dedicated to three of these areas: the location of the Brahma Granthi, the Vishnu Granthi, and the Rudra Granthi. As you learn to lock and squeeze like a yogi, you strengthen your body from the inside out.

Emotions, Trauma, and Bandhas

When engaged, bandhas recirculate prana's energy to push past blockages and stagnation in the body. Through the use of bandhas, you will learn to engage the muscles located deep within. By practicing these techniques, every muscle will begin to activate. Through this activation, buried muscles, emotions, and memories will start to emerge. This act of purification wakes up the body, allowing it to release what no longer serves your highest and best good.

This may manifest in the clearing of old emotional residue such as anger, pain, shame, and fear. Any emotion previously packed away will begin to resurface to be healed. When we choose not to engage in the internal work to heal and move past what has harmed us, we inadvertently replay the same traumatic situations in relationships and experiences throughout our lives. Most people don't choose what is best for them; they choose what is familiar. The more you lock difficult thoughts and feelings away, the longer they remain in the background, jumping and yelling, begging to be seen. What you don't own owns you. And what you don't heal, you repeat.

When you meet someone and immediately feel as though you have known them forever, most likely, you have, in the form of past relationships, wounds, traumas, and experiences. Memories, events, and emotions can get stuck in your cells, causing you to repeat the same cycles—healthy or not. Over the years, and in moments of extreme stress, knots and kinks form in the body. Think of it in terms of a clogged pipe. When a pipe is backed up and blockages become too large to allow the flow of liquid, extreme pressure is used to remove the obstruction. Much like the pressure of a plunger, band-has build up tension to push past blocks, resulting in the movement of pranic energy throughout the body.

In this chapter, we will practice each bandha individually, strengthening the relationship with these areas within the body. Mastering these techniques allows you to benefit from the kriyas ahead and to achieve the emotional freedom we each desire. It is not uncommon to be unable to feel the location of the bandhas as you begin this process. Many people have had trauma or injury to these areas, causing the surrounding muscles to "turn off" and disengage. Should this be the case, the ability to stretch, strengthen, and turn on the muscles of your pelvic floor (the location of your root lock, or Moola Bandha) may begin as a struggle.

As you start engaging your bandhas, pay close attention to the mental and emotional responses you have surrounding locking and building pressure in these areas. Particularly if you have had any form of trauma, sexual or otherwise, a medical or healthcare professional's help is recommended. As we have discussed, the body holds emotions. Cells store trauma, stress, pain, and shame, and as such, do not enter into this practice lightly. As you push past blockages, know that buried emotions and memories bubbling to the surface can be intense. Proceed gently, with loving care and mindfulness. Now that you are aware that uncomfortable feelings or emotions may surface, take care to practice bandhas cautiously and methodically, and slowly introduce these life-altering techniques.

Conscious Effort for Lasting Change

Kundalini yoga may seem slow to many, particularly in our fast-paced world. But because of the power of bandhas, you must begin delicately, using the flow of Mother Nature as a guide. Suppose you have been holding on to trauma for decades, potentially lifetimes. Would it not be irresponsible and unsafe to power through without proper preparation? There is nothing wrong with doing something simply because it is hard, but there is a time and place to push your body, and the bandhas' execution is not one. You are working with sacred energy, and it is with that knowledge you begin to engage in the practice of bandhas. Your body is a temple; your emotions are holy. Treat the entirety of your being with kindness and compassion, moving forward slowly and with intention. Pay close attention to how your body reacts and adjust accordingly.

The goal of every word and exercise in this book is for the highest and best of all. That includes your mind, body, and spirit, just as it does mine. Please, feel free to use whatever additional tools you deem appropriate to support yourself along this journey. Write in a journal, call a friend, hug a loved one, take your puppy for a walk, rest when you need rest, and seek professional medical help when your body instructs you to do so. We are all intuitive beings. If we listen closely enough, we can hear our soul's calling; our highest and best will let us know when we push past the threshold of our health and safety.

Psychic Knots

In Sanskrit, the word *granthi* means knot or doubt. Individuals who wear a sari or dhoti create a small pouch using the fabric to hold and secure money within their attire. This purse is connected via a knot and is therefore commonly referred to as a granthi. In our Kundalini practice, granthi refers to the three psychic knots within the body. It is said that the constriction of these knots blocks the path to enlightenment.

The metaphor for these blockages is best explained via a lesson from Buddha.[103] One day, Buddha brought a silk handkerchief to a meeting with his disciples. First, he showed

---

103. Saeed, "Mindfulness Is Untying the Knots."

the crowd the fabric, which was long, outstretched, and free of knots or kinks. He proceeded to pull the handkerchief, showing its malleability and length. After demonstrating its dexterity, Buddha tied five knots in the handkerchief. Buddha asked his disciples if the silk fabric, now in knots, was still the same. They responded that the rope was the same, yet different.

Buddha, acknowledging their response, explained that each of his disciples was Buddha, but they were unable to see their divinity because they were each tied and bound in knots. Buddha demonstrated the fabric's tightness with a quick tug on the handkerchief, its flexibility reduced. The fabric was more rigid, less malleable than before. As he tugged each end, he showed the crowd how the knots got tighter, not looser. Referring back to his disciples' comment, he asked, "Why do you try to open your knots by pulling?"

Buddha's lesson was that our acts of doing are often our undoing. By pulling too hard (i.e., trying too hard), we inadvertently amplify our constrictions, making the situation even more difficult to untangle.

Buddha concluded the sermon by asking his disciples what could be done to untie the knots. How could the fabric's unraveling occur when pulling and forcing it only perpetuated the bind, making the situation worse? One disciple responded that to untie the knots, attention must be paid as to how the knots came into existence in the first place. Through undoing from the inside out, the knots could be unraveled. In agreement, Buddha directed each disciple to meditate upon their knots so they could begin to excavate the root of their entanglements in an attempt to untie and lengthen.

The pulling of these knots (i.e., forcing a situation or outcome) is rampant in everyday life. The philosophies of yoga continually instruct us to surrender, but we are bombarded by the pressures of daily life. No matter how often you practice or how many hours you meditate, part of the human experience is the internal push and pull between force and surrender. When you do not address the root of an issue, it presents itself in different forms in your life. It is like taking a pill to fix an ailment instead of getting to the root cause of the symptom. So too do we tug on the ends of our ropes, unsuccessfully attempting to pull ourselves out of uncomfortable situations.

The Three Granthis

The Kundalini practice of engaging the bandhas helps unblock stagnation within the body. By paying close attention to the granthis, you take the journey further by getting to the roots of these blockages. Each psychic knot is also referred to as an emotional knot. Strive to untie or unravel each granthi so you can offer your emotions and trauma to be healed.

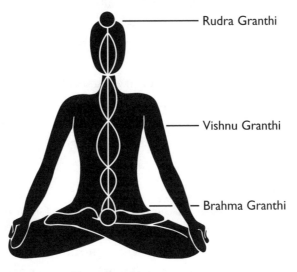

Three Granthis

Brahma Granthi

Beginning at the root, we first examine the Brahma Granthi. Associated with the Moola Bandha, this psychic knot works with the first two chakras, the mooladhara and the swadhisthana.

It is here that you store desire, particularly the urge for food and sexuality. With all passion encompassed in this region of the body, the phrase most commonly used to embody this energy is "I want."

Examining this knot's emotions from a negative perspective, this energy's misappropriation manifests itself as excessive selfishness, negativity, lethargy, and ignorance.[104] Should you catch yourself feeling any of these emotional side effects, direct your attention to this area within the body to unravel the stagnation.

---

104. "Principles of Yoga—3 Granthis."

Vishnu Granthi

Second, we introduce the Vishnu Granthi. This granthi connects to the third, fourth, and fifth chakras: manipura, anahata, and vishuddhi.

It is here that your emotions, thoughts, and expressions of self shine through. By connecting to the solar plexus, heart, and throat chakras, you express this energy as, "I want to keep."

Connected to the practice of Uddiyana Bandha, it is here that you utilize the pulling and tightening of the abdomen and solar plexus region to move the energy of Vishnu. Vishnu was known as the sustainer, and it is here that we connect with the rajas—the tendency toward passion, ambition, and assertiveness.[105]

Rudra Granthi

Lastly, we begin to understand the energy of Rudra Granthi. Rudra was dubbed "the destroyer" in the Hindu faith, and it is here that we start to destroy the need and want for all that we previously desired before the enlightenment of these higher chakras.[106] This granthi's connection to the ajna and sahasrara chakras is one of higher consciousness.

Here, you unknot the need for material possessions and unravel the thought processes that keep you from achieving your highest potential. You learn to surrender the ego. As this knot unties, you begin to understand the interconnectedness of all things, heightening your psychic awareness.

What Is a Bandha?

Bandhas, or yogic locks, are techniques to hold or tighten specific muscles within the body to recirculate pranic energy. While constricted, bandhas create a build-up of tension to push past blockages and stagnation upon their release. If psychic knots are the body's energetic response to emotion, bandhas are the physical way to untie these knots. Similar to Buddha's story, this pranic energy allows you to find your way to the center of these knots, unraveling them from the inside out. The pressure of the bandhas builds, forcing things previously hidden to the surface—hence the many warnings about taking the locking process slowly. Things are hidden for a reason, particularly the emotions associated with them. It's often easier to pack them away than address them at the

---

105. "Principles of Yoga—3 Granthis."
106. "The Granthis."

moment they occur. Bandhas are an intentional way to call forth these wounded parts of yourself so you can offer them up to be healed.

Traditionally bandhas were classified as mudras, handed down through yoga lineages via word of mouth.[107] Most pranayama and mudra techniques mention these mysterious bandhas with little instruction past "squeeze the moola bandha" or "apply root lock." Their intersectionality with the exercise's effectiveness is of great importance, but the explanation needed to perform bandhas correctly is rarely given.

This is why I have chosen to dedicate a chapter to these three techniques and the chakras they amplify. Bandhas are instrumental to a spiritual awakening; the redirection these blockages create sends all of the pranic energy into the sushumna nadi.[108] Through repetitive practice, you untie your psychic knots, redirect your life force energy, and achieve higher consciousness.

Moola Bandha

We begin with the Moola Bandha for the same reason we first spoke about the Brahma Granthi: This root lock connects with the two lower chakras. As the location of sexuality, safety, and security, this foundational position propels energy up through the sushumna nadi and each of the remaining chakras. Allow me to briefly remind you that the sushumna nadi is one of the three most important nadis because it runs along the spinal column, intersecting with more than 72,000 nadis and all seven chakras.

By beginning at the root, we clear the foundation, pushing pranic energy upward to clean out all stagnant energy.

Associated with survival instincts and the desire to procreate, this primal energy is the foundation of the chakra pyramid. Located at the base of the spine, the Moola Bandha prevents the downward flow of energy from exiting the body via the lower gates. (The gates refer to the locations of exit and entry in the body.) Should negative emotions surrounding your most primal instincts and needs leave the body, you inadvertently dump your life force, full of negative vibrations, into the ether or into another person. But the knot is still intact, acting as an internal generator and multiplying this energy from your most sacred regions. Over and over again, the cycle continues. The knot tightens, releasing these emotions out of your lower extremities. Attempting to remove unwanted

---

107. Satyananda Saraswati, *Asana Pranayama Mudra Bandha*, 471.

108. Satyananda Saraswati, *Asana Pranayama Mudra Bandha*, 471.

feelings is futile, for the knot will continue to tighten and pulsate with agitation until you find the courage to address the root and heal.

Although not always stated, it is advised to apply Moola Bandha at the end of yoga postures to increase their effect. Similarly, it is almost always advised to apply a light neck lock in seated postures and many other asanas.

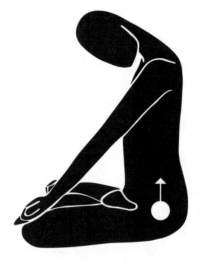

Moola Bandha

As you engage the Moola Bandha, you change the direction of this energy. Instead of giving away your power, you take it back and redirect this energy within. You no longer choose to do what is easy by pushing away or numbing your emotions. Instead, you decide to face and work through them. You engage the root lock, pulling your pelvic floor up and in, with self-love. It is as if you are saying, "I am worthy of love. I am worthy of security. I deserve to feel safe and supported in my body." You decide to no longer look for another to provide safety and security. With each lock, you say to your highest self, "I am here for us. I choose us. We are no longer dependent on others for our foundational needs. We are safe. We are supported. We are loved."

When you come to acknowledge the power of your energy—your prana, your life force—you begin to harness the ability to heal yourself. Each Moola Bandha works to soften this lower knot ever so slightly so that one day, you truly will feel your emotions transmute as they no longer cause you pain and suffering.

The Moola Bandha does more than work through what binds you. Located just above your dormant Kundalini energy, it is vital to actively practice Moola Bandha in order to open the gate, allowing your Kundalini energy to move. Unlocking this energy center is said to allow the Kundalini energy to rise and not fall back down. Akin to "getting out of your own way," as you heal these fragmented pieces of yourself, you pave the way for your highest, most abundant, and most authentic self to take the wheel. Your primal urges and emotions no long run the show. The more you practice Moola Bandha, the lowest of the three locks, the more you consciously experience all of the benefits of security and sexuality.

Uddiyana Bandha

Uddiyana Bandha is the second of the locks, located up the spine near the abdomen. We are intentionally discussing these in order, for as you will see in Maha Bandha, the sequence of this engagement is vital for effectiveness and safety. It is by moving methodically up the spine that we work to unblock the pathway to enlightenment. Until you reach the anahata, or heart chakra, you have not experienced a full Kundalini awakening and your Kundalini energy is just as likely to fall, descending back to the base of your spine, dormant again. Work with the technique of Uddiyana Bandha to untie the second knot to allow your Kundalini energy to rise freely. Without its unlocking, this energy will continue to rise through the Brahma Granthi and perpetually fall back to its dormant resting place.

Associated with the second knot, Vishnu Granthi, the implementation of Uddiyana Bandha activates the manipura and anahata chakras. The manipura is located in line with the navel at the solar plexus. The anahata aligns with the area of your heart. Uddiyana Bandha's motion activates by pulling the navel deeply toward the spine, in and up, to engage this lock. The movement of pulling the navel inward activates the solar plexus chakra, while pulling upward activates the heart chakra. With the engagement up and in, the two chakras are simultaneously connected in one motion, combining their energy and recirculating prana throughout this entire region. This exercise is incredibly beneficial for overall digestive health because this area is the location of the majority of the body's digestive organs. The recirculating of prana in this region clears toxins and debris, making way for Kundalini energy to rise.

Through the practice of Uddiyana Bandha, you gain control over your emotions and your gut's response to them. There is a reason your gut is referred to as your second brain.

Emotions are often felt physically in the abdomen before they are intellectually acknowledged. The gut reaction you have to circumstances can "tie you up in knots." The moment you feel any form of emotion in your abdomen, you can work with this bandha to relieve the discomfort by actively pushing your breath's clearing qualities through the area to detoxify and transmute the energy. Feeling emotions is not the concern; it is the act of holding on to these emotions that wreaks havoc on the physical body. With the brain-gut connection directly linked through this bandha, you begin to release the feelings migrating to this region as soon as they occur.

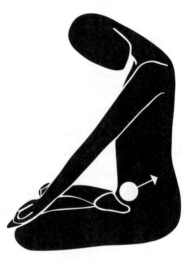

Uddiyana Bandha

Jalandhara Bandha

The highest of the three, this bandha is associated with the Rudra Granthi, the third of the granthi knots. Commonly called throat lock, the Jalandhara Bandha is located at the fifth chakra, vishuddhi. The throat chakra is the location from which we "speak our truth." Regardless of the lower two bandhas' simultaneous engagement, the engagement of this bandha will provide courage and improve your ability to express yourself clearly. As the throat chakra clears through this lock's activation, the two uppermost chakras are also activated.

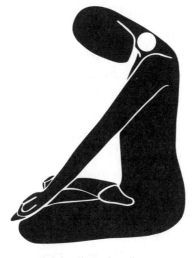

Jalandhara Bandha

Until this point, Kundalini energy has ascended with the potential of falling and lying dormant once again. Using the Jalandhara Bandha to unlock the Vishnu Granthi allows this energy to move upward into the heart chakra. Once the Kundalini energy passes the heart chakra and into the throat, the area activated first through Jalandhara Bandha, the path to enlightenment clears. With intentional effort, the Kundalini energy will continue to rise without the possibility of it rescinding below the heart chakra. Continual work is required to coax this energy further upward, but once you begin the action of untying the Rudra Granthi, the higher functions of enlightenment begin to appear.

This knot's untying moves upward through the chakras, from vishuddhi, the throat, to ajna, the third eye, and finally sahasrara, the crown. As you move through vishuddhi, you are empowered to use your voice, no longer bound by doubts or constrictions that kept you from speaking your truth. At ajna your intuition heightens, creating a clear path to see the truth in any situation. When your Kundalini energy finally reaches sahasrara, you move to a place of direct communication with the divine. As you ascend, you are no longer bound by physical, mental, and emotional attachments. Your intuition heightens, and you are able to drop the physical ailments holding you back. It is here where a singular idea reshapes itself into one with a more universal impact. Your thoughts change from "me" to "we," focusing on healing the collective instead of healing only yourself. You begin to use your voice, your throat chakra, to speak out against injustices through this unlocking, bringing the darkness into the light.

Kundalini Rising

Kundalini energy is represented as a serpent coiled three and a half times at the base of the spine. Each technique used in Kundalini's practice works with the subtle energies within the body to unblock and remove all stale and stagnant energies so that you make way for your Kundalini to rise. Located just below your root chakra, this energy ascends from your spine's base up through the seven chakras and more than 72,000 nadis in order to reach samadhi. Samadhi is the highest form of enlightenment or consciousness that one can achieve while still in the physical plane, or in an earthly body.[109] It is in this state that we are said to experience continual, pure bliss.

Pulling together the teachings of this chapter, we understand how the intersectionality of these techniques aids in the awakening of this Kundalini energy. Intrinsic muscles squeeze to perform the Moola Bandha, Uddiyana Bandha, and Jalandhara Bandha, placing pressure on the three granthis. By learning the bandha's techniques above, you utilize the energy of your breath to create a building pressure against these three psychic knots. As you release these constrictions, the pressure against the blockages retracts, resulting in a forceful release of energy that opens the knots. With this opening, what was previously stuck begins to dislodge and is swept away through the breath's continual action. This is how to clear the path for your Kundalini, but you must take care to actively work through the released emotional stagnation in order to ensure that these knots remain unblocked so Kundalini energy can continue to ascend.

Kundalini Awakening and Extrasensory Gifts

I was taught that Kundalini energy resides within the causal body. This is the area of one's aura, which extends one foot from your physical form in all directions. It is within this space that you interact with and feel the energy of others.

As you tap into the powers of your Kundalini energy, your ability to assess people and situations will accelerate. The nonverbal cues of others become more pronounced; you become more in tune with your emotional landscape, and therefore the dynamic landscapes of others. You might find that you pick up on the feelings of others regardless of their physical proximity because your Kundalini energy can unlock your psychic powers as it unties the psychic knots.

---

109. *Encyclopaedia Britannica Online*, s.v. "Samadhi," updated Februrary 17, 2021, https://www.britannica .com/topic/samadhi-Indian-philosophy.

As your Kundalini rises, the ability to expand your aura outward increases. This means that your energy field intertwines with the energy field of others at any given moment. If, during this expansion, you do not actively put energetic boundaries in place to protect yourself, this stimulus can be overwhelming. Modern spirituality calls this the act of "waking up"—similar, if not identical, to a Kundalini awakening.

As we have discussed, a Kundalini awakening is not a path for the faint of heart. All that you uncover must be dealt with, for once you know, you cannot unknow, just as once you see, you cannot unsee. This is why you need to proceed methodically and with cautious intent, for "waking up" will be difficult, and "waking up" too fast can be downright dangerous.

Cautions for a Kundalini Awakening

The likelihood that anyone reading these words will fall victim to the "dangers" of a Kundalini awakening is not likely, but it is important to discuss nonetheless. We live in an age where technology is abundant and being overstimulated is the norm. In extreme situations where one might renounce everyday life and voyage to the outskirts of society in order to search for spiritual pursuits, the dangers of a Kundalini awakening are genuine. The teachings in this book are to aid you in your Kundalini awakening in a way that is natural and that fits with modern society, not in a way that renounces it.

The cautions around awakening your Kundalini energy most often refer to the impatience of the human condition. As humans living in a modern world, unlocking your Kundalini is intensified by the mounting to-do lists and pressures of everyday life. Like the desire to achieve a corner office your first year out of school, the haste to achieve one's goal often results in the urge to skip a plethora of necessary steps. But just as you must learn to build a foundation in your professional life, so too must a foundation be built in your spiritual practice. Each chapter in this book is designed to build upon another in order to create that solid foundation, which will support you not just today, but throughout this lifetime and into the next.

I do want to be clear that Kundalini's energy is immensely high flying, and if you are someone who lives the majority of your time with your head in the clouds, pay close attention to how your Kundalini practice affects you. I myself have had to dial back my Kundalini practice on many occasions when I found myself ungrounded and unable to move through the pressures of modern life with my feet firmly planted.

Kundalini is said to "get you high naturally," and the ancient texts speak of those who have gone mad when their Kundalini awakened too quickly. I myself have witnessed the instability of the beginning stages of this phenomenon twice, once in India and once in the states. It is very important to mention that both of these individuals were actively partaking in drugs of other kinds. Because I witnessed the less-than-ideal combination of drugs and a deeply spiritual ascension practice, I do not suggest the use of such extra-curricular activities, plant medicine or otherwise. I say this as a nod to your safety, not from a place of judgment about how you choose to live or experience life. I want nothing more than your highest and best, and in order to move through your Kundalini journey both effectively and safely, I suggest that you first experience Kundalini in its purest form before you add additional stimuli to the equation.

To further calm any potential fears of danger, it is instructed that the preparation for a full Kundalini awakening is not something that will occur in one lifetime. It is a journey that a soul actively prepares for with each incarnation. One could argue that as I am writing a book on this topic, my soul has been on this journey long before I inhabited this body in this physical plane. You may or may not have a guru or a desire to move to an ashram, as the Vedic texts suggest, but since we are here, together, at this moment, it is clear that you do have a desire to awaken your awareness. Awakening your Kundalini energy is not the end game. As that reality sinks in, allow your shoulders to soften away from your ears. You are here to utilize this energy in order to make modern life a little more palpable and enjoyable. The knowledge and exercises that follow will allow you to do just that.

Exercises: Squeeze Like a Yogi

The following exercises help you in your journey to squeeze like a yogi. You will learn how to engage these intrinsic muscles in the most subtle and effective of ways. Pay close attention to how your knowledge of these energy centers alters your Kundalini experience moving forward. How does being both conscious of their effect and conscious of your intent to activate them translate into a heightened awareness of the subtle energies present in every other area of your life?

⟶ *Technique* ⟵
Moola Bandha (Root Lock)[110]

Cautions: Refrain from aggressively performing Moola Bandha during the menstrual cycle.

Duration: One minute.

Posture: Sit comfortably in an easy pose or lotus pose with a straight spine.

Drishti: Eyes gently close as the internal gaze focuses on the third eye.

Technique: To engage Moola Bandha, envision the sex organs contracting and tightening. This action contracts and releases the pelvic floor, reducing the circumference of negative space in these regions. Focus on the constriction at the perineum.

Action: Continue briefly contracting and relaxing this region, feeling the center of your pelvic floor move up and in as the muscles engage.

Repetition: As you begin, the muscles that regulate the contraction and relaxation of the anus and urinary passageways will also contract. Continue to practice breathing naturally until your awareness increases and you are capable of only constricting the muscles in the mooladhara region.

Checking the Technique: Perform Moola Bandha by engaging the muscles of the pelvic floor, pulling them up and in. At first, you may notice that your pelvis rocks, tilting backward. The cue to engage Moola Bandha is up and in, not back and up. Should you find your pelvis rocking, simply realign, stacking your spine squarely on top of your pelvis and pulling the muscles up toward your spine.

Benefits: Aids in the stimulation of the pelvic nerves, which can help tone the urogenital and excretory regions. Redirects energy to the sushumna nadi, aiding in a spiritual awakening.

---

110. *Moola* = Root, firmly fixed, source, cause.

∽ *Technique* ∼
Uddiyana Bandha (Abdomen Lock)[111]

Cautions: If suffering from disorders such as colitis, ulcers, diaphragmatic hernias, heart disease, glaucoma, or increased intracranial pressure, this bandha should be avoided.[112] Avoid if pregnant.

Duration: One minute.

Posture: Sit comfortably in an easy pose or lotus pose with a straight spine. The arms stretch straight. Actively press the palms against the knees.

Drishti: Eyes gently close, and the internal gaze focuses on the third eye.

Technique: Inhale fully, filling the body with a full yogic three-part breath, followed by a full yogic three-part exhale. On the completion of the exhale, contract the abdominal muscles inward and upward. Utilize the pressure of the hands, the straight arms, and the shoulders to provide a solid base for the lock's concave action to occur.

Action: Inhale fully, exhale fully, and then perform Uddiyana Bandha. To begin, hold the breath for five seconds before releasing the retention. Upon release, the shoulders, arms, neck, and head soften.

Repetition: Begin with three rounds, gradually increasing the rounds and the retention duration over time.

Variations: Uddiyana Bandha is most commonly performed in a comfortable seated position but can also be performed standing, slightly bent over with the hands actively pressing against the knees. You will not be capable of performing this technique on a full stomach, as the body will be engaged in digestive functions and unable to contract fully.

Checking the Technique: You will notice that your abdomen will become more concave as your ability to expel all air from your body increases. Visualize pulling this up and in behind the rib cage, creating the look of a deflated soccer ball in the abdomen.

Benefits: Aids in the stimulation of the pancreas and helps with liver function. Massages the internal organs, which can improve overall organ health. Helps balance the adre-

---

111. *Uddiyana* = To rise or fly upward.

112. Satyananda Saraswati, *Asana Pranayama Mudra Bandha*, 481.

nal glands, which can reduce lethargy as it improves blood circulation of the torso. Can improve digestion and reduce unwanted belly fat.

⌒ *Technique* ⌒
Jalandhara Bandha (Throat Lock)[113]

Cautions: Anyone suffering from cervical spondylosis, intracranial pressure, vertigo, high blood pressure, or heart disease should not practice throat lock.[114]

Duration: One minute.

Posture: Sit comfortably with the legs crossed and the knees firmly in contact with the floor. Hands rest on the knees.

Drishti: Eyes gently close, and the internal gaze focuses on the third eye.

Technique: Inhale slowly, holding the breath in retention after the inhale. As you hold the breath, tilt the chin downward, locking the chin against the neck. Curl the tip of the tongue up and back, pressing it against the roof of the mouth in Khechari Mudra. The arms stretch straight, locking the shoulder, elbow, and wrist joints in place. The shoulders hunch forward and upward, aiding in the arms' locking.

Action: Inhale deeply, applying throat lock on the retention. Hold the retention, engaging all of the body's muscles. Gently release on the exhale and slowly raise the head and neck, relaxing the shoulders down the back.

Repetition: Begin by holding your breath for five seconds. As you strengthen your stamina in this posture, extend the length of the retention and the number of times you practice the full cycle of breath: inhalation, retention, and exhalation.

Variations: Jalandhara Bandha can be performed with retention after both inhalation and exhalation.

Checking the Technique: The first few times you practice this technique, you might notice the energy redirecting toward the shoulders. The constricting of the neck can be incredibly uncomfortable, especially if you have a thyroid condition or have trouble

---

113. *Jalan* = Net. *Dhara* = Stream or flow.

114. Satyananda Saraswati, *Asana Pranayama Mudra Bandha*, 474.

speaking your truth. Take care not to exhale or inhale until the full lock is released, including the chin, arms, and shoulders.

Benefits: Can relieve sinus pressure, improving overall sinus health. Can decrease the heart rate and relieve stress, anxiety, and anger. Can help balance thyroid function.

⎯ *Technique* ⎯
Maha Bandha (The Great Lock)[115]

Cautions: Avoid if suffering from cervical spondylosis, intracranial pressure, vertigo, high blood pressure, or heart disease. Avoid if pregnant.

Duration: One minute.

Posture: Sit comfortably in an easy pose or lotus pose, with spine straight and palms pressing against the knees.

Drishti: Eyes gently close, and the internal gaze focuses on the third eye.

Technique: A full inhale is followed by a full exhale, removing all air from the body before beginning retention. Engage all three of the bandhas (Moola, Uddiyana, and Jaland-hara Bandha) in order, contracting from the bottom up.

Action: Take care to engage the locks in order, moving from the bottom up: Moola Bandha first, Uddiyana Bandha second, and Jalandhara Bandha third. The locks are released differently than the order in which they were engaged. Uddiyana Bandha is released first. Next, Moola Bandha is released, followed lastly by Jalandhara Bandha.

Repetition: With each lock, focus your attention on the area of constriction. Begin with three rounds, increasing both the rounds and the retention duration progressively over time. Only increase the number of rounds after you feel you have perfected the act of one full inhalation, exhalation, and then retention.

Checking the Technique: Direct your attention to the areas locked in the wavelike manner. If you are having trouble feeling the constriction of these areas, avert your attention to other areas of the body that might be attempting to compensate for these actions. Are your hips gripping or shoulders tightening to aid the posture? Are your feet flexing

---

115. *Maha* = Great.

or neck muscles straining past the point of constriction, toward pain? Observe these constricted areas, then soften and re-center your gaze to the task at hand.

Benefits: Aids in regulating the entire endocrine system, which can increase sexual health, abdominal functions, and thyroid regulation.

✑ *Technique* ✑
Maha Bheda Mudra[116]

Maha Bheda Mudra is qualified as a lock mudra, as it combines mudras with bandhas. As we learned, utilizing the Maha Mudra encompasses using all three bandha locks to circulate the body's pranic energy.

Cautions: This technique must be executed on an empty stomach in order to engage the locks effectively. Avoid if suffering from cervical spondylosis, intracranial pressure, vertigo, high blood pressure, or heart disease. Avoid if pregnant.

Duration: Three minutes.

Posture: Begin sitting with the legs elongated, weight resting on the tailbone and hands at the sides. Bend the left knee and press the heel of the left foot into the location of the perineum, or mooladhara chakra. With the right leg straightened in front of the body, place both hands on the right knee. After the exercise completes with the left knee bent, switch the legs, performing the same movements with the right knee bent.

Drishti: Eyes gently close, the internal gaze focused on the third eye.

Technique: Sitting with an erect spine, the left foot tucks under the body as the right leg outstretches. Deeply inhale. On the exhale, lean forward with a long spine, interlacing the fingers around the right big toe.

Action: As you grasp the toe with the fingers, inhale with a long spine, tilting the head slightly back. Fold forward on the exhale, hold the breath at the bottom of the exhale, and perform root lock, Moola Bandha, and throat lock, Jalandhara Bandha. The abdomen will be in Uddiyana Bandha naturally due to the full exhale and forward fold.

---

116. *Maha* = Great. *Bheda* = Piercing. *Mudra* = Gesture or attitude.

Repetition: One full inhale and exhale with retention is one full round. Move through each leg for a full breath. Hold the retention as long as you can, extending the breath's length with each round.

Modifications: If your flexibility level does not permit you to reach the toes, modify by bringing the hands further up the legs to the top of the feet, ankles, calves, or shins, depending on your physical limitations. Take care to keep the foot flexed, regardless of the hand position. If needed, utilize a strap to engage the feet and the hands.

Checking the Technique: All three bandhas (the root lock, abdomen lock, and throat lock) are engaged. The arms remain lengthened throughout the practice, as does the spine.

Benefits: Aids in regulating the entire endocrine system, which can increase sexual health, abdominal functions, and thyroid regulation.

ᔒ *Technique* ᔒ
Three-Minute Har

Duration: Three minutes.

Posture: Sit comfortably in an easy pose or lotus pose with a straight spine. A light Jalandhara Bandha is engaged.

Mudra: Fingers extend straight, gently pressed against one another.

Mudra I: Hands connect at the Jupiter side, palms facing downward, the thumbs crossing below the hands with the right thumb under the left.

Mudra II: The hands separate, palms turning inward in a circular motion, closing the circle by connecting the side of the pinky fingers at the moon mound, hitting the alternate side of the hands together.

Drishti: Eyes soften and are 90 percent closed. Gaze focuses on the tip of the nose.

Mantra: "Har" is chanted externally.

Technique: With the elbows bent, the hands come together at the center of the chest. The first movement begins with the Jupiter side of the hands connecting, right thumb crossing below the left. The mantra is chanted when the hands are connected and when the hands circle to connect the pinky fingers on the moon mound. The mantra is again chanted when the hands circle back to their starting position, right thumb crossed under the left. The motions complete a circle at the heart center.

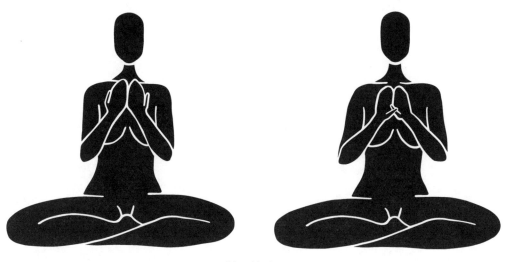

Har Mudra

Action: Connect the hands on the Jupiter side, right thumb under the left. The hands move away from one another, connecting on the moon side, palms facing up with the side of the pinky fingers touching. The mantra "har" is spoken out loud on the impact of the moon side and the Jupiter side.

Repetition: Repeat this motion, combined with chanting one "har" per second on impact, for three minutes.

Checking the Technique: "Har" is chanted with the tongue's tip, tongue flicking the upper palate. Pull the navel in with each chant of the mantra "har." Chant "har" as you hit the Jupiter side of the hands, palms facedown, and the moon side, palms faceup.

Benefits: Can enhance prosperity, bringing wealth and abundance into your life.

Ten

Sing Like a Yogi
(Utilizing the Vibration
of Mantras)

IN RELIGIONS THROUGHOUT THE world, singing hymns or reciting prayers is an integral part of devotional practice. I have fond childhood memories of Sunday mornings in church, waiting with bated breath for the next hymn to be sung. The hymnal perched on my lap, open to the correct page. Ever the prepared student, I was ready to belt out the lyrics at the top of my lungs. My childlike amazement had no concept of the words and lessons being put forth. All I knew was that I loved it. It was fun, cathartic even, and easily my favorite part of the service. As I matured, I came to understand the verses' meanings. Their words hit me on a different level with each new passage of life. I innately understood the power of song, especially devotional songs sung as a collective. This practice was an integral part of my religious upbringing, though that did not stop me from feeling utterly out of place the first time I attended a Kundalini yoga class.

The first time I entered a room filled with individuals wearing all white, we were invited to recite invocations in unison. As the chanting began, everyone seemed to know the words and heed their meanings, singing in perfect unison. I was uncomfortable, as many of us are the first time we try something new. *What are they saying, and how do they know how to pronounce the words correctly? Does everyone know the meaning of these chants but me?* My mind was so distracted that I failed to lean into how the words and unified experience made me feel.

How was this any different from standing shoulder-to-shoulder with my Jewish friends and family as they recited Hebrew prayers on a high holiday? Wasn't the experience similar to the countless dinners I had with my European family, where the conversation continually shifted between English, French, and Italian? Had I not gazed with admiration as I witnessed devout monks chant during their daily rituals or respectfully observed my Muslim friends perform their daily prayers?

Yoga, up until that moment, had been a form of exercise for me, a way to release stress and strengthen my body. It had somehow never occurred to me that yoga might also be, just as equally, a connection to the divine. The mantras I heard recited that day were the first of many. I was unsure of what occurred, though when I released control and allowed myself to sink into the experience's vibrations, the sounds touched me on a cellular level. To this day, when practicing with a large group of people, I feel the vibrations deep in my soul with each mantra repetition. It is as if the cobwebs within my body are being shaken loose from the inside out.

What Is a Mantra?

Mantras are sacred sounds, vibrations that help open the mind to connect to the divine, the Universe, and the highest and most pure version of ourselves. The working with and chanting of mantras is an intentional experience. We release control of what "should" happen, vowing instead to be present during what *does* happen. The simple act of choosing to engage in the recitation of a mantra is one of surrender. It is a surrender to the ego, because you no longer worry if you look silly doing it. It is a surrender to the dialogue of your rational brain as you recite words that are likely not of your native tongue. With surrender, your need to understand and rationalize the experience temporarily subsides.

The beauty of mantras is that once you experience the practice, surrender your need to control, and focus on feeling instead of rationalizing the effects, you may now use it as a stepping stone for all other experiences in your life. Not only do you have tools to bring you back to that meditative state, but you also have a stable baseline for how surrendering control of the mind and leaning into faith has served you, no matter how scary the experience was. Mantras do not just help you—they create profound results in every aspect of your life.

The Vibration of a Mantra

As you feel into the energy of a place, person, or thing with good "vibes," you are tapping into the vibration of the experience. Imagine a tuning fork. As you tap the fork, visualize the sound waves vibrating through the ether. This is what occurs when you recite mantras. Mantras create vibrations, rattling the neurons in the body. Just as the sound waves of a tuning fork create vibrations strong enough to move small particles of dirt and soil visibly, so do the recitations of mantras. When people recite together in unison, they amplify the vibrations, using the power of sound waves to unearth the stuck places within themselves. You can almost feel the dirt shifting loose and sifting through the body as the mantra cleans you from the inside out.

Every time you make sound waves with your words, you evoke a vibrational frequency. You alter energy through sound, and that sound changes your energetic makeup at a cellular level. You have probably witnessed the ripple effect of skipping a stone across a pond. Just as you see the vibrational frequencies created by tapping a tuning fork or skipping a rock, a shift in perspective changes your awareness surrounding the internal effects that occur as you chant. Once you correlate the cleansing vibrations in the body with the external energetic effect of reciting mantras, it becomes obvious why these practices occur across all demographics and religions: The effects of mantras are palpable.

The effects of chanting mantras increase with one's intent. Throughout this book, I have spoken openly and repetitively about the importance of intention when performing all components of your spiritual practice. When praying with mantras, the intent behind the prayer amplifies the affirmation's effect. Prayer in the form of chanting mantras lives in the vibration of faith. Faith helps people move forward to achieve or accomplish their objectives.[117] With the invocation of mantras, you lift your mind, body, and heart to Source in the act of intentional faith. By chanting mantras, you simultaneously raise your vibration and strengthen your faith.

Mantras and the Subconscious

We each have an internal monologue looping from our subconscious. The energy behind these thoughts has a tangible effect on the matter both around and within you whether or not these thoughts are verbalized. Your inner dialogue is creating a vibrational ripple

---

117. Ishwardas Chunilal Yogic Health Center, *Prayer and Mantrajapa*, 2.

effect inside you. This isn't as easy to see as the ripple effect from a stone skipping across the pond, but it is easily felt.

The power of the mind can take the lead and control virtually every avenue of your existence. The vibrations you create amplify harmonious and disharmonious interactions with yourself and your surroundings. Vibration is matter, so the vibrations you create, create matter. Whether you are speaking your truth or pendulum-swinging toward the side of negativity, the words you speak create a ripple effect throughout the world. This ripple affects you externally and internally.

I want to clarify that it is the cause and effect of your subconscious vibrational thoughts that cultivates your experiences. Though "speaking things into existence" is a logical interpretation of the yogic science behind mantras, simply saying something does not make it true nor inevitable. The recitation of mantras places you in a meditative state. While in this meditative state, you are capable of accessing the subconscious. It is here that the vibrations of a mantra take root. Merely speaking negative or positive thoughts out loud does not result in negative or positive experiences in your life. When you control your thoughts, you are capable of deep healing and growth. Mantras help you access the root of your programmed beliefs by using their vibrations to shake up the paradigm, and this can create lasting, authentic change.

Chanting Mantras Is an Inside Job

It is said that spirituality is an inside job. As you dive into mantras, you will begin to feel the effects of this inside work immediately. The sayings take on tangible feelings and emotions as this practice becomes a regular part of your life. When you begin to utilize mantras, it is common to think of this new process as singing toward something. For example, a deity at the front of the room, a teacher upon their meditation pillow, or your ancestors or loved ones. This resonates intellectually as sound and vibration leave the body, moving out and away. But how does your experience shift when you direct the vibration inward, first and foremost?

As you begin to incorporate the knowledge that vibration is matter and realize that the vibrations of your thoughts and actions internally scrub your being and your external environment, you should begin to look at the practice of mantras as an internal shower. As learned in the previous chapters, the methods of pranayama scrub intrinsic debris from the body. Referring once more to the visualization of a tuning fork, the vibrations of mantras also clean the inside of the body in a similar way. The breath uses oxygen to move stagnation, while mantras use vibration. Through the unsticking of unwanted particles, mantras cleanse all that no longer serves you. Mantras free the debris from its sticking place so that the breath may wash it away.

The energy of mantras is subtle. Small shifts occur within that cause you to show up differently in your everyday life. Others may comment on this shift, but the transition is so subtle that you may not be able to pinpoint precisely what has changed. Yet, if your mantra practice is rooted in dedication and intention, you will immediately know what shift they are referring to.

Mantra Yoga

As one of the seven types of traditional yoga, mantras are a practice all their own. The seven types of yoga are diligently studied at universities as students obtain knowledge from the ancient scriptures. As we begin to embark on the path of mantra recitation, let's discuss the concept of japa meditation, or *Mantra Japa*, the recitation or chanting of a mantra.[118]

Stages of Mantra Japa

When learning a mantra, it is important to listen to pronunciation, rhythm, and meaning. There are three steps to chanting a mantra:

1. Vaikhari Japa: Spoken out loud; emphasis on precise, correct pronunciation

2. Upanshu Japa: Whispered; chanted softly with an open mouth in a meditative state

3. Manasa Japa: Mentally recited; chanted with the lips sealed, creating an internal vibration

First, chant the mantra out loud. The emphasis in this initial step of Vaikhari Japa is the correct pronunciation of the words. Traditionally, this chanting is done loudly in order to practice and strengthen proper pronunciation. After the phrase's pronunciation has been practiced and learned, move on to Upanshu Japa. Here you begin to recite the mantra in a soft, whispered tone. Focus begins to move internally as you speak the words. The third and final of the stages is Manasa Japa, when the mantra is chanted internally.

---

118. *Japa* = Recitation.

As you practice japa, you strengthen the muscle of your mind. Understanding the progression as taught through the Vedic scriptures can be used to enhance your inner awareness as you progress through the stages. These stages, facilitated in this order, increase your ability to concentrate. You calm the mind while maintaining a level of alertness throughout the practice. If you have tried to recite mantras internally without the disciplined practice of stages one, Vaikhari, and two, Upanshu, there is a strong possibility that you found yourself fighting the desire to fall asleep as you skipped ahead to stage three, Manasa. Without the mental agility gained by performing steps one and two, the difficulty of step three, Manasa, may cause the brain to shut down, particularly if you are already fatigued.

The practice of mantras is just like all other components of yogic science. To set yourself up for success, begin slowly, each technique compounding upon the other. Cut yourself a little slack if you have struggled with mantras in the past. If you began to nod off the first time you sat in silence, chanting a mantra silently, no worries! This is why you must actively practice the progression of the prior techniques. Yoga is a series of methods that build with each interaction. And remember, yoga is a practice. It gets better with time! Each day unveils new hurdles and challenges, but you reap tremendous rewards with each mountain overcome.

The Most Famous of All Mantras

OM is the sacred sound of the Universe. One of the seven beeja, or seed mantras, OM represents the collective consciousness. It is further explained as the sound heard throughout all time and space: the primordial sound, or primary vibrations of nature. OM, also written as *Omkar*, is nature's pulse, evoked with each recitation of the mantra.

Without explanation, the pronunciation of OM can feel a little tricky. If you have attended a yoga class where the room's energy was grounded, opened, or closed with this invocation, you might have experienced the disharmonious attempts of multiple individuals striving to match one another's tone and pitch. Though experiences like this might feel off-putting at first, once you learn how to move your mouth—and what sounds accompany those movements—the entire process becomes a little less scary and a little more harmonious.

How to Pronounce OM

OM is pronounced A-U-M.

- A: Feel the vibration of A deep within the abdomen
- U: Feel the vibration of U move up through the body into the lungs and heart
- M: Feel the vibration of M through our head and brain

To begin OM's sound, first take a deep inhale, filling the abdomen, chest, and clavicle with air. Open your mouth to an O shape, allowing the sound "Aaaaaaaa" to come out of the O-shaped mouth as you exhale. Take your time.

The "Aaaaaaaa" sound continues to be made as your mouth naturally begins to decrease the circle's size. When the O shape is reduced by half, you will begin to notice that the sound naturally changes from "Aaaaaaaa" to "Uuuuuuuu."

The sound of "Uuuuuuuu" vibrates as the O shape continues to reduce in size, making the final sound of "Mmmmmmmm" as the lips touch.

As you practice this mantra in its three traditional parts, you will begin to notice the differences in vibration as the A, U, and M sounds are emphasized. It is also important to note the proportions of the three parts of A, U, and M. The first sound, A, is made for three seconds, followed by another three seconds of U. The final sound of M lasts three to four times as long as the first two, extending between nine and twelve seconds. The entire sound of A-U-M lasts between fifteen to eighteen seconds in total.

If you find it difficult to chant OM for the entire fifteen seconds, take note of where you are chanting from. Without a full yogic breath—filling first the abdomen, then the chest, and finally the clavicle—you will not have enough oxygen to last the entire fifteen seconds. Engage the entire body's power by using a full yogic breath, focusing on each of these three parts as you chant. Release the air first from the abdomen chanting A, next to the chest as you chant U, and from the clavicle as you chant M.

OM in Practice

To fully integrate this shift in pronunciation from OM to A-U-M, practice the difference in the enunciation of the O and the M in OM versus the A, U, and M in A-U-M.

Begin sitting in a chair or on the ground in an easy pose. Sit with the spine upright. The shoulders roll back and the neck lengthens. Envision pulling the center of the ears in line with the center of the shoulders. The center of the shoulders aligns directly over the centerline of the hips. Actively reach the crown of the head toward the ceiling, lengthening both the neck and the spine. Begin with a deep inhale, filling the lungs from the lower abdomen. Allow the lower belly to fill, inflating the stomach outward as the pelvic floor drops and air begins to rise from the belly to the lungs. The chest cavity fills, expanding the ribs outward, and the breath eventually reaches the throat.

As you exhale, begin to make the sound of "Oooooooo." Hold this sound as the breath leaves the body, switching to "Mmmmmm" as the breath is released halfway. The sound "Mmmmmm" is made with the lips pressed together as the breath continues to descend, leaving the second half of the body. This is a two-part breath. The O sound is made for the first half of the exhale, and the M sound is made during the second half. How large was the mouth when the O sound began? Did the transition to M feel natural or forced? Did you have to consciously think about switching from O to M halfway, or did the switch occur organically? Where did you feel the vibrations? In your mind? Throat? Belly? Try this exercise a few more times, leaning into how the sound makes you feel. Does it feel natural and fluid? If not, what does it feel like?

When you're ready to try this with A-U-M, begin the same way. With the spine straight, shoulders relaxed, and neck long, begin to fill the abdomen with air, following the previous cues. On the exhale, start by making the "Aaaaaaaa" sound through an O-shaped mouth. As the mouth starts to close approximately halfway, begin to make the sound "Uuuuuuuu." The "Uuuuuuuu" sound continues as the mouth closes, reaching the sound "Mmmmmmmm" as the lips press together. This is a three-part breath. How large was the mouth when the A sound began? Did the transition to U feel natural? What about the transition from U to M? Did you have to consciously think about switching from A to U to M, or did the switch occur organically? Where did you feel the vibrations? How did this differ from the experience of chanting the mantra OM as an O-M two-part breath? Repeat the exercise a few more times, focusing on these questions to hone your technique.

Was the experience of A-U-M considerably more pleasant than OM? Did it feel more organic? How will this change your experience moving forward?

Seed Mantras

With the correct pronunciation of OM firmly rooted in your practice, we will now learn the beeja, or seed mantras. Each seed mantra, including OM, correlates directly to one of the seven chakras. Because they are capable of invoking the chakras' energy as they are chanted, seed mantras are said to be charged mantras. They are mantras that quite literally plant the seed for insurmountable change. You will notice that each of these mantras also follows the musical scale.

Similar to OM's chanting learned above, each of these seed mantras is spoken with a long, drawn-out vibration, phonetically closer to Lllllllaaaaaaammmmmm than the three simple letters of "Lam." By using these mantras, you realign the chakras and tap into the energies they empower. In the previous exercise, you explored the vibration of A-U-M versus OM in your body. The remaining seed mantras are felt internally in the same way. As you chant the mantra for each chakra, feel the vibration of this invocation within your body. Focusing on the chakra in question amplifies the pulse, creating a multidimensional experience as the mantra is chanted with the right pitch. At the same time, focus your drishti on the specific chakra with the intent of invoking its energy. Envisioning the chakra color adds another layer of purpose, compounding the healing effect of your practice.

To chant the mantras on key, run through the musical scale, starting at the base of your spine with the root chakra mantra "Lam." As you ascend the spinal column, you will hear the tone progression up the scale. To further enhance your ability to pronounce the mantras correctly, implement a technique called *solmization*, which originated in ancient India. Solmization is assigning syllables to the different "steps" of the scale.[119] If you are familiar with the movie *The Sound of Music*, utilize its famous do, re, mi melody to warm yourself up for this practice. This movie adaptation of solmization brought this technique into the modern age, and it can help put these mantras into practice correctly.

Chakra Number	Chakra Name	Chakra Color	Mantra	Note	Syllables
7	Crown	Violet	OM (AU silent, M out loud)	B	Ti
6	Third Eye	Indigo	OM (AU out loud, silent M)	A	La
5	Throat	Blue	Ham	G	Sol

---

119. Kovalchik, "Why Are Notes of the Tonal Scale Called 'Do, Re, Mi,' etc.?"

Chakra Number	Chakra Name	Chakra Color	Mantra	Note	Syllables
4	Heart	Green	Yam	F	Fa
3	Solar Plexus	Yellow	Ram	E	Mi
2	Sacral	Orange	Vam	D	Re
1	Root	Red	Lam	C	Do

Begin implementing these mantras just as you did in the OM exercise. Sit with your spine straight, the crown of the head reaching toward the ceiling, and the shoulders back. Instead of your drishti on the third eye, turn this gaze to the mantra's chakra. As you shift the focus to the chakra's location, envision the sound swelling's vibration at its center. The experience deepens as you visualize the pulse growing. Continue to strengthen this meditative state by imagining the chakra's color expanding outward from its center as you chant. Imagine the mantra's vibration amplifying the color from the center of the chakra out into the Universe.

As you chant, the forming of words creates different frequencies. Those vibrations and the relationship between the tongue and the mouth stimulate other portions of the brain. Depending on your state of mind at the time of these mantras, the experience will vary drastically. With each small change in your physical, mental, or emotional state, you show up differently. Regardless of how you arrive, the intent is always the same: to cultivate a relationship with your higher self. Just as your emotions ebb and flow, so too does your relationship with your practice. Each time you chant, you enter into the experience as a new person, and you exit forever changed.

Exercises: Sing Like a Yogi

The following exercises will help you sing like a yogi by invoking the sacred sounds of the Universe. Through the use of mantras, these sacred vibrations will shake off the cobwebs of your soul, aiding you in manifesting your soul's greatest desires.

⌒ *Technique* ⌒
Antar Naad Mudra Meditation

Duration: Eleven minutes.

Posture: Sit comfortably in an easy pose with a straight spine.

Mudra: The pinky fingers bend in toward the palms, touching the tips of the thumbs. The remaining three fingers extend straight. The arms extend straight as the backs of the hands rest against the knees.

Drishti: The eyes close as the gaze focuses internally on the third eye.

Mantra: "Sa Re Sa Sa. Sa Re Sa Sa. Sa Re Sa Sa Sa Rung. Har Re Har Har. Har Re Har Har. Har Re Har Har Har Rung."

Technique: The mantra is chanted with the arms and fingers straight and outstretched from the body as the back of the hands rest on the knees. Sit bones press firmly on the floor and the head's crown actively reaches toward the ceiling, creating a straight spine.

Action: Focus the gaze on the third eye. Hold arms and spine straight as the mantra is continuously chanted.

Repetition: Repeat the mantra for eleven minutes, then meditate.

Checking the Technique: The arms and first three fingers actively outstretch in a straight line down and away from the center of your body. As you straighten your limbs, envision your spine actively lengthening in opposition.

Benefits: Aids in the removal of negativity and opens the chakras. It is said that anyone who practices this meditation is granted prosperity, creativity, and protection against attack.

⌒ *Technique* ⌒
Meditation for Protection and Projection from the Heart

Duration: Eleven minutes.

Posture: Sit comfortably in an easy pose with a straight spine.

Mudra: The palms press together with the pointer, middle, ring, and pinky fingers touching one another. The thumbs are crossed.

Drishti: The eyes close. Focus the gaze on the third eye.

Mantra: "Ad Guray Namay. Jugad Guray Namay. Sat Guray Namay. Siri Guru Dayvay Namay." [120]

Technique: Begin with the hands at the heart center.

Action I: While chanting the first line, "Ad Guray Namay," the hands move slowly away from the body at a sixty-degree angle. The extension of the arms occurs throughout the line, ending with straight arms as the last syllable of "Namay" is sung.

Action II: Inhale, bringing the hands back to heart center.

Action III: As you sing the next line, "Jugad Guray Namay," the hands move slowly away from the body at a sixty-degree angle. The extension of the arms occurs throughout the line, ending with straight arms as the last syllable of "Namay" is sung.

Action IV: Inhale, bringing the hands back to heart center.

Action V: The extension of the arms away from the body continues as the third line, "Sat Guray Namay," is sung. The hands move slowly away from the body at a sixty-degree angle. End with straight arms as the last syllable of "Namay" is sung.

Action VI: Inhale, bringing the hands back to center.

Action VII: As the last line, "Siri Guru Dayvay Namay," is chanted the hands move slowly away from the body at a sixty-degree angle. The extension of the arms occurs throughout the line, ending with straight arms as the last syllable of "Namay" is sung.

Repetition: Repeat the mantra for eleven minutes, then meditate. If you feel so called, you can increase the duration of this technique in five minute increments, eventually extending it a maximum of thirty minutes.

Checking the Technique: Movements are slow and controlled as if moving intentionally through water. The movement of the mudra away from and back toward the body is

---

120. *Ad Guray Namay* = I bow to the primal wisdom. *Jugad Guray Namay* = I bow to the wisdom through the ages. *Sat Guray Namay* = I bow to the true wisdom. *Siri Guru Dayvay Namay* = I bow to the great unseen wisdom.

fluid. There is a brief pause before the next line of the mantra is sung. As the hands move away from the body, envision a bright, white light of energy opening and expanding the heart. With each recitation of the mantra, the heart opens further and a white shield of light extends from the center, protecting your auric body.

Benefits: Aids in creating a protective shield of white light energy that surrounds the body.

∽ *Technique* ∽
The Morning Call

Duration: Eleven minutes.

Posture: Sit comfortably in an easy pose with a straight spine.

Mudra: The hands are in Gyan Mudra. The backs of the hands rest on the knees.

Drishti: Eyes gently close with the internal gaze focused on the third eye.

Mantra: "Ek Ong Kar. Sat Nam Siri. Wahe Guru." [121]

Phonetically: Ek Onnng Kaaar. Sat Naaam S'ree. Wha-hay G'roo.

Technique: Sit comfortably in an easy pose with the fingers in Gyan Mudra. The spine is straight, the crown of the head reaches toward the ceiling, and the chin is fixed in a neck lock.

Action I: As you inhale deeply, vibrate a short "Ek" as you pull in the navel. Then exhale, chanting "Ong" and letting it vibrate in the sinus cavities before transitioning to "Kar" for the rest of the breath. The sound is continuous; do not pause as you transition from Ong to Kar. Take care to vibrate both Ong and Kar at the mouth's upper palette and then through the nose, giving equal time to them both.

Action II: Inhale deeply, chanting "Sat" as you draw in the navel. On the exhale, chant "Nam" until you are almost out of breath. Siri (S'ree) is spoken quickly at the last moment before the breath expires.

---

121. *Ek* = One. *Ong* = Creator. *Kar* = Creation. *Sat* = Truth. *Nam* = Name/identity. *Siri* = Great. *Wahe* = Beyond description. *Guru* = Dispeller of darkness, teacher. Read more at Shakti Parwha Kaur Khalsa's "My Favorite Mantra."

Action III: Instead of another long deep breath, begin with a short half breath for the mantra's last part. On the exhale, start by breaking Wahe into two syllables, Wha-hay. The pronunciation of Guru (G'roo) is slightly drawn out. The end of this three-part mantra runs together as almost one syllable: hayg'roo.

Repetition: Repeat the mantra with eyes softly closed and palms resting gently on the lap for eleven minutes. Upon completion, inhale deeply, focusing your attention on the third eye. Hold the breath at the top of the inhale, re-center your internal gaze, exhale, and relax. Meditate.

Checking the Technique: This mantra is an ashtang mantra, meaning it is a mantra of eight syllables. Though there are eight words in the mantra, the pronunciation instructions listed above delineate where to extend the words. Combine them properly to execute the eight syllables. As you progress through this mantra, you may notice your tone dropping. Observe and tune back in to the vibration, remembering to keep the neck lock applied and head upright.

Benefits: Aids in opening and balancing the chakras, which can create a direct connection between you and the divine. Stimulates Kundalini energy.

◟ *Technique* ◞
Healing Meditation to Help Those in Need

Duration: Eleven minutes.

Posture: Sit comfortably in an easy pose, spine straight.

Mudra: The elbows are tucked tightly against the ribs. The elbows are bent, forearms extending from the center of the body at a forty-five-degree angle. The palms are open and flat, facing up. Wrists are pulled back, fingers together and thumbs gently spread. Consciously make sure your palms are flat.

To make the palms flat, bend your wrists almost to the point of hyper-extension. As you do this, feel the wrists, palms, forearms, and biceps activate. Begin to envision the healing energy emitting from your palms toward the person(s) you are sending this white light energy to.

Drishti: The eyes close. Mentally visualize the person(s) you wish to send healing energy to. Apply neck lock.

Mantra: "Raa Maa Daa Saa Saa Say So Hung." [122]

Technique: Sit comfortably in an easy pose with flat palms. The spine is straight, the crown of the head reaches toward the ceiling, and the chin is fixed in a neck lock.

Action I: Inhale and chant the mantra, one repetition per breath. Pull the navel in sharply when pronouncing "Hung" to keep yourself from holding the sound.

Repetition I: Repeat the mantra for eleven minutes, paying attention to the movement of the mouth and feeling the resonance of each sound in the mouth and sinus area.

Action II: Deeply inhale. Hold the breath, envisioning the person(s) you wish to send healing energy toward, and engulf them in healing white light. Exhale.

Repetition II: Repeat the healing visualization for three full breaths.

Action III: Deeply inhale. Raise the arms to the ceiling, vigorously shaking the upper extremities. Arms remain in the air on the exhale.

Repetition III: Repeat the upper extremity energy release for three full breaths.

Checking the Technique: As you recite the first Sa and Hung, pull the navel firmly inward. With Hung's recitation, the last syllable ends forcefully as the navel pulls deeply toward the spine.

Benefits: Aids in sending healing energy to those near and far. Stimulates Kundalini energy. Can increase physical energy levels.

⌒ *Technique* ⌒
Meditation for Elevation, Connection, and Joy

Duration: Eleven minutes.

Posture: Sit comfortably in an easy pose, spine straight.

Mudra: Hands rest on the knees with the palms facing up. The tips of the pointer finger and the thumbs connect in Gyan Mudra.

Drishti: Eyes soften, focusing on the tip of the nose.

---

122. *Raa* = Sun. *Maa* = Moon. *Daa* = Earth. *Saa* = Impersonal infinity. *Saa Say* = Totality of infinity. *So* = Personal sense of merger and identity. *Hung* = The infinite, vibrating, and real.

Mantra: "Ang Sang Wahe Guru." [123]

Phonetically: Ung Sung Wha-hay G'roo.

Technique: Sit comfortably in an easy pose with hands in Gyan Mudra. The spine is straight and the crown of the head reaches toward the ceiling.

Action I: Deeply inhale. Begin chanting the mantra.

Repetition I: Repeat the mantra for eleven minutes. Eyes are focused on the tip of the nose and hands rest gently in the lap in Gyan Mudra.

Action II: Deeply inhale. Hold the breath and apply root lock. Drishti moves to the third eye. Envision joy filling up the entirety of your being. Exhale.

Repetition II: Perform the inhale, hold, and exhale three times. Then meditate.

Checking the Technique: Are you straining with the eyes, hips, hands, fingers, or arms? Have your shoulders tightened? Add softness to the postures, chanting the mantra with a sense of interconnectedness and joy.

Benefits: Can activate the seventh chakra, which can strengthen the connection to one's highest self and help with feelings of unity and humility. Can activate radiance, interconnectedness, presence, and protection.

∽ *Technique* ∽
The "Last Resort" Meditation

Duration: Eleven minutes.

Posture: Sit comfortably in an easy pose, spine straight.

Mudra: Place your hands in your lap with the palms facing up. The right hand rests in the left. The tips of the thumbs are touching.

Drishti: Eyes gently close, internal gaze focused on the third eye.

Mantra: "Wahe Guru Wahe Jio."

Phonetically: Wha-hay Guroo, Wha-hay Guroo, Wha-hay Guroo, Wha-hay Jee-O.

---

123. *Ang Sang Wahe Guru* = The Infinite Being, God, is with me, and vibrates in every molecule and cell of my being. Read more at 3HO's "Meditation for Elevation, Connection, and Joy."

Technique: On a long, slow exhale, chant the mantra eight times.

Action: Take a deep breath in, slowly releasing the breath as you chant the mantra in a monotone voice.

Repetition: Repeat the mantra for eleven minutes, eyes softly closed and palms resting gently on the lap.

Checking the Technique: The exhalation will take approximately forty-five seconds for the mantra to be chanted all eight times. If you find it challenging to complete the mantra without running out of breath, stop, breathe out and in, and begin again.

Benefits: Can promote relaxation, strength, and mental clarity.

⟳ *Technique* ⟲
Shabad Kriya

Duration: Eleven minutes.

Posture: Sit comfortably in an easy pose, spine straight.

Mudra: The hands rest in the lap with the palms facing up. The right hand rests in the left. The tips of the thumbs are touching and pointing forward, away from the body.

Drishti: The eyes are 90 percent closed, gazing down at the tip of the nose.

Mantra: "Sa, Ta, Na, Ma. Sa, Ta, Na, Ma. Wahe Guru."

Technique: Sit comfortably in an easy pose with the hands resting in the lap. The spine is straight and the crown of the head reaches toward the ceiling. Before adopting the mudra and beginning the kriya, tap the finger alongside the thigh while chanting the mantra, gaining confidence in the mantra's prescribed cadence.

Action I: Inhale the breath, repeating the mantra "Sa, Ta, Na, Ma" in four rhythmic counts. Each of the four parts is chanted internally at equal intervals for a total of four beats.

Action II: Hold the breath. As the breath is held, the mantra "Sa, Ta, Na Ma" is internally counted for four rhythmic counts. Do this four times for a total of sixteen beats.

Action III: Exhale for two counts, mentally chanting "Wahe Guru," for a total of two equal beats.

Repetition: Repeat the mantra for eleven minutes.

Benefits: Can promote relaxation, which may aid in the regulation of the pineal gland, promoting hormonal balance. Beneficial to perform before bed to promote a night of rhythmic sleep.

Eleven

Practice Like a Yogi
(Kriyas to Amplify Intentions)

WE'VE REACHED THE END of our journey. With the fundamentals of Kundalini yoga understood and the techniques executed, you are ready to tackle your Kundalini practice. As you learned in chapter 1, a kriya combines postures, mudras, mantras, and bandhas to create the desired result. The intention behind the actions is what sets kriyas and Kundalini yoga apart from other types of yoga. Kriyas balance the elements and chakras, and each Kundalini kriya is crafted with a particular outcome in mind. Kundalini kriyas boast titles such as "Breath of Fire" and "Ego Eradicator." These are pointed, self-explanatory names, clearly stating the intended result. Like all other yogic endeavors, these techniques are laid out through intent, cadence, and progression.

This final chapter is an example of such an intention. Each previous direction was methodically placed in an order and sequence. The knowledge and experience you have built compound to this crescendo. With Kundalini's science explained and executed in the previous chapters, we can now focus on fine-tuning your practice. This chapter will set you up for success by ensuring that you have all the tools in your yogic tool belt that are needed to create an enjoyable and sustainable Kundalini experience from this day forward.

Tuning In

In the lineage of Yogi Bhajan, before each class begins, it is customary to chant the Adi Mantra three times. The Adi Mantra is "Ong Namo Guru Dev Namo."[124] Also referred to as "tuning in," it is this beginning invocation that signifies the start of class. It is a mutual agreement between the physical and spiritual planes to begin. The chanting of Ong Namo grounds the room's energy, bringing attendees to the present moment and syncing their vibrations with one another.

This mantra connects you to the teachers that have come before you. The purpose of a Kundalini practice is to connect with the infinite wisdom of the Universe. It is through this chanting that practitioners communicate their willingness to begin. This mantra is thought of as a way to open the door to connection with the masters, teachers, and loved ones that came before us, and to the divine teacher within. It is chanted three to five times.

If you are new to chanting mantras, this practice might feel uncomfortable. If chanting mantras makes you feel uneasy, try saying them internally. The vibrations you create may not ripple outward through your mouth, but they will vibrate internally, creating an equally important effect. The intention behind the mantra is what is most important. By pushing past the feeling of discomfort, you further open your heart. It is the belief in something greater than yourself, as well as something greater within yourself, that aids in moving through this fear. Open your mind and heart to communication with a higher power and the divine teacher within.

The Importance of Daily Practice

The previous chapters taught that yoga builds upon a backbone of structure and discipline. Kundalini yoga energetically builds upon itself, compounding its benefits with each repetition. A daily practice has life-altering effects, even if you only practice for three minutes a day. In my practice, I have found that a few short minutes every day creates more significant results than an extended session once a week. Kundalini's repetition can strengthen the immune system, heighten intelligence, and open the heart. The energetic benefits are so profound that regardless of the kriya's length, you will begin to witness immense shifts in all areas of your life.

---

124. *Ong Namo Guru Dev Namo* = I bow to the creative wisdom; I bow to the divine teacher within. Read more at 3HO's "Kundalini Yoga Mantras."

I suggest beginning with a three-minute exercise, committing to practice it every day for the next twenty-eight days in the same location at the same time. This repetition of time, duration, and place further amplifies the kriya's effects. By harnessing a lunar phase's energy, you allow the body to experience the full range of emotions this practice brings forward. And as you slowly work through a three-minute kriya, you cultivate the body's opportunity to shift, creating a space for these changes to occur on a cellular level. Kundalini is a physical practice, but the real magic lies in the shift within the energetic body.

In the Kundalini tradition, it is essential to choose a meditation that calls to you and practice it for forty days. By committing first to twenty-eight days with the intent to make it to forty, you break down the endeavor into smaller milestones, setting yourself up for success. Once practicing for twenty-eight days becomes a breeze, forty days feels like a much less arduous task. Earlier in this book, you learned that forty days is the proverbial "top of the mountain" when the subconscious begins to take over and the cellular makeup of the body starts to change. This cellular change is what creates lasting effects on the mind, body, and soul.

Regardless of how attuned you are to your physical body, energetic shifts can feel extreme and overwhelming. Dipping your toes into this practice by creating a safe space to experience this transformation is another way of honoring your soul's path. Repetition of the same exercise in the same location at the same time each day recirculates this energy of transformation. It allows you to be divinely supported in your pursuits as you reaffirm your love for yourself each and every day.

Kundalini Flu

As you work to create lasting change, you practice Kundalini with the intent of permanently modifying your body through this change on the cellular level. Kundalini, a method of unblocking, removes stuck or unwanted energy. Through the use of Kundalini techniques, you work to remove all that no longer serves you. The ultimate goal is to create a container of balance and equilibrium where you function as the most authentic and whole version of yourself.

If a Kundalini awakening occurs too quickly, the emotions and experiences previously dormant may rush to the surface in a manner that may feel overwhelming. This same phenomenon occurs when someone who lives on fast food and sweets switches to a diet of predominantly fruits and vegetables. The fiber and detoxifying properties of a whole-food, plant-based diet begin to unclog decades of calcified toxins in the body. Symptoms like headaches, chills, and body aches might present as the body works over-time to remove unleashed toxins. A similar experience can occur during the practice of Kundalini—years of calcified, dormant emotions are released into the system to be cleared from the body.

New age culture coined the phrase *Kundalini flu* to describe the body's physical response to this energy release. Potentially presenting as aches, pains, chills, or lethargy, these symptoms are not unique to Kundalini, as the phrase suggests. Flu-like symptoms can occur when any form of deep energy work is done. Modalities such as acupuncture and Reiki can cause similar effects as energy is unblocked. Just as the body works to expel a virus, so does the body remove repressed feelings and emotions that are unlocked during Kundalini's practice.

As you move energy via movements and meditations, by-products are produced that need to be expressed and released. Tearing up or crying is natural; so is swaying. Getting chills or having involuntary jerks or trembles might also occur. If you know this before-hand, you can begin to challenge thoughts about how your practice "should" look, which allows you to remove judgment from yourself and others.

Yoga Etiquette

During a Kundalini experience, never touch others without their permission. This rule of keeping your hands to yourself translates to every area of life, particularly during the sanctity of any deeply personal spiritual work. Yoga creates a sacred space for all to feel safe and welcome. The moments of emotional and physical unblocking that Kundalini generates can present externally. This might confuse the person practicing and/or those around them. Seeing your neighbor in pain, or even experiencing great joy, may make you want to reach over to comfort or embrace them, but by doing so, you may inadvertently interrupt their healing. Our bodies are profoundly capable of healing themselves. Though reaching out feels like a knee-jerk reaction of kindness, this is a moment when you must tap into your yoga training and execute the power of the pause.

Instead of reacting, utilize the wisdom of a deep breath. Take this moment to think through your next steps so you can react from a position of strength. Because of Kundalini's repetitive structure, you have the mental fortitude to pause, breathe, and process a situation before moving forward. Similar to being proactive instead of reactive, sometimes that extra second or two is all that you need to ride the brief emotional wave of your triggers. Taking a second to re-center keeps you from saying or doing something you might otherwise regret.

If you feel the uncontrollable urge to hug someone after class, ask first. Practicing Kundalini together will create feelings of intimacy for people you barely know, potentially compelling you to physically share that affection. This is another excellent opportunity to practice honoring boundaries and cultivate the power of the pause. Even the most physically affectionate person may not want to be touched after a vulnerable experience. Practice holding yourself and your fellow yogis with love and kindness by honoring their individual experience and, unless you have permission, keeping your hands to yourself.

Sharing Sacred Space with Others

Entering into a collaborative practice with someone you love is a beautiful thing. The compounding benefits can skyrocket your connection to a new level of intimacy, but it is beneficial to open communication channels before you proceed. Discussing how you wish to show up on your mat sets the stage for an open and respectful experience for you both. Talking through what you have learned about how your physical and energetic body may respond to Kundalini will prepare you for what might occur as a united front.

Practicing Kundalini yoga with a loved one can be an incredibly spiritual experience, but let's not forget that even the most intimate relationships require healthy boundaries. Purposely letting another into such a sacred space is an expression of trust. The vulnerability it takes to welcome someone into the depths of your heart and soul in this way is often the impetus for change, producing a closeness not found through other avenues. The key to this is, once again, intention. The intention to let in another. The choice to be vulnerable. The will to surrender control and let the Universe guide not only you, but your partner as well.

This agreement between your souls is a two-way street. This contract is one that honors and respects the individual you are in partnership with and yourself. Your body feels different every day, as do the bodies of those around you. Communicate your level of physical comfort often and in advance. When you wait to express yourself until you are at a breaking point, healthy boundaries turn into walls to block others out. Begin to think of how you might desire comfort, or lack thereof, before and after your practice. Communicate that need the moment it occurs, and communicate every time your desires change. Kundalini provokes constant change, and the ability to communicate these fluctuations with someone you cherish opens avenues of conscious conversation in all other areas of your life.

Closing Practice

It is now time to introduce Kundalini's traditional closing invocations. There are two mantras used to end class, utilized differently depending on which lineage of Kundalini you perform. During my studies of traditional Kundalini in India, I practiced the mantra "Om Shanti." While studying Kundalini in the States, I became familiarized with the mantra "Sat Nam." As you customize your Kundalini practice, I suggest giving both mantras a try.

Choose the invocation that resonates with you most sincerely and practice it for the next forty days. In the forty days that follow, implement the second mantra. At the end of this eighty-day cycle, choose the mantra that connected with your solar plexus and stirred up something within your soul. Select that mantra and stick with it.

As your body restructures and your energetic field clears, be open to the possibility that your connection with your chosen mantra might change. Should that happen, give yourself permission to be fluid. All journeys have ups and downs. What worked for you in one season of your life may no longer resonate as you enter another. Recommit to yourself and your practice every day. The deeper the connection with yourself grows, the easier it will be to discern what—if anything—you need to change, and how to do so.

Om Shanti

In the teachings of traditional Kundalini, the recitation of "Om Shanti" is used to signify the end of practice. Just as we learned to chant Ong Namo three times to begin class, so too is Om Shanti chanted three times at the end. The word *Shanti* means peace, and its meaning alters slightly with each recitation. First, you offer up peace to yourself, then to those around, and finally, to the world:

Om Shanti, Shanti, Shanti = Peace to myself, peace to all who surround me, peace to the world.

Sat Nam

A similar invocation is utilized in Yogi Bhajan's lineage of Kundalini through the phrase "Sat Nam." Sat Nam is a beeja, or seed mantra, meaning it is chanted in one syllable. Pulling from Yogi Bhajan's Sikh heritage, the word *Sat* is extended as it is sung (Saaaaat), ending with an emphasis on the T. The letter is spoken as the tongue touches the teeth. Nam is expressed similarly (Naaaaammmmm), drawing out the A and M to close.

   Sat Nam = Truth is my identity.

Covering the Eyes

I was taught that at the end of one's practice it is customary to rub the palms together, then to cover the eyes with the palms before they open. During your Kundalini practice, a continuous loop of energy is created within the body. As you move, chant, meditate, and squeeze, you work to build and strengthen the body through this energetic re-circulation. The act of covering the eyes before they open places the energy created into the body instead of allowing it to escape from the palms or eyes.

   To perform this loop-closing technique, rub the palms together aggressively while the eyes remain closed. This creates a magnetic field between the hands. Next, cup the hands over the eyes so that all corners of the palms and fingers touch the face. The fingers squeeze together to block out any remaining light. When you open the eyes, they will widen into full darkness, absorbing the magnetic energy created by the palms. The eyes are two of the nine gates of the body, believed to take in and expel energy. Still deprived of light, rotate the eyes clockwise in one full circle, then counterclockwise. This allows the energy to reach the entire surface of the eye, ensuring maximum absorption. Shut the eyes again behind the palms, closing this technique by bringing the hands back to prayer posture at the heart center. Complete your final dedications, prayers, chants, words of gratitude, etc. Finally, open your eyes as your practice is completed.

Coming Home to Yourself

As we close out this text, we come full circle. We are all seeking, searching, learning, and growing daily. As you embark on your journey toward knowledge and truth, you will become sidetracked by the ebb and flow of life. It's common to be tricked into thinking that the next great thing, which is just around the corner, will change everything. Happiness is that new job, house, partner, child, pet, body… The list goes on and on. These triumphs bring instantaneous joy, but the shine begins to fade as you strive toward your next goal. Regardless of the time between your successive victories, the more you dedicate yourself to the inner work of a practice like Kundalini, the more you begin to realize that accomplishments are not what brings happiness.

Happiness begins within you. It is an innate truth that we are each born with goodness, hope, and light. You live each day with internal divinity, cultivated and reinforced through your actions. By committing daily to yourself, you reaffirm your resolve to love, honor, and cherish the soul. The relationship you cultivate with yourself is what you are seeking. In each of those external triumphs, you look to come home to yourself. Kundalini is a medium to nurture this relationship. It takes work—hard work—as all things worth achieving do. Some days you soar through your practice in a meditative state of bliss. Other days you curse yourself, the method, and everyone in earshot, overwhelmed by the wave of emotions coming to the surface. In the moments of highs and lows, the most important thing is that you continue to show up. You show up for yourself. The secret sauce behind this practice is discipline and intention. Without one or the other, you will falter. With both, you can do nothing but soar.

One of the best things about yoga, regardless of the lineage, is that it is always different. Even if you perform the same flow, breathwork, mantra, or sequence every day, it will feel different each time. Every time you step onto your mat or meditation pillow, you show up as a completely new version of yourself. That day's trials and tribulations are different from the day before. What came quickly yesterday might be unbearable today. And though it can be utterly frustrating at times, there is a feeling of great peace in this understanding: No matter how far you come, there is always farther to go. The road (or mat) rises to meet you where you are today. Wherever you go, however far you roam, Kundalini will always be there to support you.

Exercises: Practice Like a Yogi

The following exercises are a cumulation of your practice thus far. By first practicing the techniques individually, you have created a familiarity within your body. The muscle memory strengthened throughout this journey will allow you to drop into a meditative state more easily as you proceed. By combining multiple techniques throughout this book, you will continue to activate the sacred centers of your being and, in the exercises that follow, you deepen the journey back home to yourself.

⤳ *Technique* ⤲
Kundalini Flu Bath

The symptoms of the Kundalini flu may leave you feeling tired, achy, and sore. Add a relaxing soak to the bath to aid in the body's detoxification process. The following soak adds minerals that are crucial for overall health and function back into the body.

Epsom salts, which are traditionally used for pain relief of sore muscles, do much more than merely reduce swelling and inflammation. Chemically, Epsom salts break down into magnesium and sulfate when diluted in warm water. Magnesium, the fourth most abundant mineral in the human body, is involved in over six hundred biochemical reactions.[125] Even with a healthy diet, most people are not consuming enough magnesium, making the addition of the pure magnesium flakes in this soak imperative for overall health.

Baking soda aids in the body's ability to detoxify by boosting circulation and encouraging its natural ability to heal.[126] This mineral addition allows the body to remove all that no longer serves it while adding in minerals that will improve bodily functions long after the soak is complete.

Cautions: Drink plenty of water before and after the bath to ensure adequate hydration, which helps with the body's detoxification ability. Refrain from adding essential oils to this soak as they could interact with the body's natural hormonal function. The purpose of this bath is to encourage the body's innate ability to heal itself and bring it back to a state of homeostasis.

Ingredients:
- 1 cup Epsom salts
- 1 cup magnesium flakes
- ½ cup baking soda

Directions:
1. Add ingredients to a bathtub filled with warm water. Allow the ingredients to dissolve.
2. Submerge your body in the water, soaking for 11–22 minutes.
3. Drain the water. Then rinse your body in a quick cold shower.

---

125. Spritzler, "10 Evidence-Based Health Benefits of Magnesium."

126. Cronkleton, "What Are the Benefits of a Baking Soda Bath, How Do You Take One, and Is It Safe?"

Benefits: Aids in detoxification, which can promote hormonal balance, increased vitamin and mineral absorption, and increased muscle and bone strength.

~ *Technique* ~
Ego Eradicator

Cautions: If you are pregnant or on the first three days of your menstrual cycle, replace Breath of Fire with long, deep inhales and exhales.

Duration: One minute.

Posture: Sit comfortably in an easy pose with a straight spine and the lips gently pressed together.

Mudra: The four fingers fold down, the pads of the fingers pressing onto the mounds at the base of the fingers. The palm is stretched wide. The thumbs stretch away from the hands and point straight up. The arms reach to the sky in a high V shape, creating a sixty-degree angle.

Drishti: Eyes gently close as the internal gaze focuses on the third eye.

Technique: With the arms firmly stretched into the air, begin Breath of Fire, rapidly inhaling and exhaling through the nose.

Action I: The arms are raised toward the ceiling, creating a high V shape. With a rapid inhale, allow the belly to fill with air, extending forward. Rapidly exhale, pulling the belly button in and up toward the spine.

Repetition I: Repeat Breath of Fire, quickly inhaling and exhaling, for one minute.

Action II: Slowly inhale, filling the entire body with air as the eyes remain closed. Hold the breath, allowing the tips of the thumbs to draw together. With the breath held and thumbs touching, release the fingers from the palms, straightening the fingers toward the sky. Hold your breath as the arms remain straight and locked tight. Engage root lock, actively pulling the sex organs inward, circulating the energy internally. Hold the breath.

Repetition II: Take one long deep breath in as the arms move upward. When the thumbs touch, draw one last sip of breath, actively stretching the arms and fingers as long as possible. While in this position, hold the breath for as long as can be sustained.

Action III: Slowly release the breath, simultaneously releasing the arms. The arms are released in an arc, creating a circle around the body as they slowly descend.

Repetition III: Repeat Ego Eradicator for one minute. The practice ends with the backs of the hands resting gently on the legs. Meditate.

Checking the Technique: As you stretch your arms up, ensure they are locked tight. Feel all of the muscles in the arms tighten, including the fingertips and hands. Release any tension in the lower extremities and soften the hips. After the arms raise into the air, take a deep inhale and exhale, allowing the shoulders to relax. Then retighten the arms without tightening the shoulders toward the ears.

Benefits: Can reduce negative thought patterns, purifies the respiratory system, and brings the hemispheres of the brain into alertness.

∽ *Technique* ∾
Meditation to Heal Addictions

Cautions: Clench your molars with enough force that you feel movement at the temples, but do not clench hard enough to create pain in the jaw or damage the teeth.

Duration: Three minutes.

Posture: Sit comfortably in an easy pose with a straight spine.

Mudra: The fingertips curl into the palms as the thumbs extend outward.

Drishti: The eyes gently close as the internal gaze focuses on the third eye.

Mantra: "Sa Ta Na Ma."

Technique: Raise the hands toward the head, placing the pad of each thumb on the sides of the temples. The palms face the forehead, curled fingers hovering an inch in front of the body. Clench the jaw, bringing the back molars to touch. With each clench, the area below the thumbs will move. The touching of the molars is not overly aggressive; it is only firm enough to feel something move underneath the pads of the thumbs.

Action: Clench the jaw together for four counts: Sa (press the back molars together and release), Ta (press the back molars together and release), Na (press the back molars together and release), Ma (press the back molars together and release).

Repetition: Repeat the corresponding mantra, pressing the molars together for three minutes. The motion will be rhythmic, molars pulsing in sync with the sounds of the mantra. Then meditate.

Checking the Technique: Adjust your hands to ensure the majority of the pad of the thumbs presses against the temples. When you clench your jaw, do you feel the temple move more so under your left thumb or your right? Do you need to adjust the placement of your hands to feel the movement evenly, or are you clenching the right side or left side of your jaw more firmly? Play around with the placement of your hands, thumbs, and the sides of your jaw until you feel pressure evenly in your mouth and underneath the thumbs.

Benefits: Can disrupt addictive and negative thought patterns.

∽ *Technique* ∽
Magnificent Mantra

Cautions: If pregnant, breathe gently and make sure to avoid aggressively pulling the navel up and in toward the spine.

Duration: Eleven minutes.

Posture: Sit comfortably in an easy pose with a straight spine.

Mudra: Place the elbows at the sides of the body and bend them so that the hands are front of the shoulders. Palms face foreward and fingers are open and relaxed.

Drishti: The eyes gently close as the internal gaze focuses on the third eye.

Mantra: [127]

Mantra	Translation
Har Har Har Har Gobinday.	God, the one who sustains us.
Har Har Har Har Mukunday.	God, the one who liberates us.
Har Har Har Har Udaray.	God, the one who uplifts us.
Har Har Har Har Aparay.	God, the one who is infinite.

---

127. "The Mantra Toolkit."

Mantra	Translation
Har Har Har Har Hariang.	God, the one who does everything.
Har Har Har Har Kariang.	God, the one for whom grace is done.
Har Har Har Har Nirnamay.	God, the one who is nameless and desireless.
Har Har Har Har Akamay.	God, the one who is all by itself.

Technique: The navel pulls in toward the spine on each "Har" as the hands close into a fist with the thumb outside and open. The R sound in "Har" is pronounced with the tip of the tongue reaching the roof of the mouth just behind the front teeth. On the inhale, between chants, the belly releases and the fingers close. On each singing of the mantra, the hands will open and close four times for each Har's repetition. As the fifth and final word is chanted, the palms open wide, remaining open until the singing of the three-syllable word is complete.

Action I: The arms remain stationary and engaged throughout the exercise. Begin chanting.

"Har Har Har Har Gobinday." The hands open and close four times, remaining open as Gobinday is sung.

"Har Har Har Har Mukunday." The hands open and close four times, remaining open as Mukanday is sung.

"Har Har Har Har Udaray." The hands open and close four times, remaining open as Udaray is sung.

"Har Har Har Har Aparay." The hands open and close four times, remaining open as Aparay is sung.

"Har Har Har Har Hariang." The hands open and close four times, remaining open as Hariang is sung.

"Har Har Har Har Kariang." The hands open and close four times, remaining open as Kariang is sung.

"Har Har Har Har Nirnamay." The hands open and close four times, remaining open as Nirnamay is sung.

"Har Har Har Har Akamay." The hands open and close four times, remaining open as Akamay is sung.

Repetition I: Repeat for nine minutes.

Action II: Deeply inhale. Hold the breath at the top of the inhale. Engage root lock, pulling the navel in as the tip of the tongue comes to the roof of the mouth and the fingers activate. Exhale.

Repetition II: Repeat two more times for a total of three rounds.

Checking the Technique: The arms remain in alignment with the midline of the body. Imagine that the body is sandwiched between two panes of glass. Strive to keep the upper extremities in between these glass panes throughout the entirety of the practice.

Benefits: Aids in creating a golden or divine protective shield. Can bring good luck and prosperity. Helps prevent self-sabotage.

～ *Technique* ～
Subagh Kriya

There are five parts to this exercise. They can be practiced for equal amounts of time, either three minutes or eleven minutes. Only part I of Subagh Kriya can be practiced as its own kriya.

Duration: Eleven minutes.

Posture: Sit comfortably in an easy pose with a straight spine.

Part I

Mudra: Fingers extend straight with an open palm, creating one long line of energy as all fingers press against one another. The thumbs are apart and relaxed.

Drishti: The eyes soften, 90 percent closed, as they gaze at the tip of the nose.

Mantra: "Har" is chanted externally, one repetition per second.

Technique: With the elbows bent, the hands come together at the center of the chest, palms facing up and pinky fingers touching.

Action: The first movement begins as the hands connect on the Jupiter side, the right thumb crossing under the left as the pointer fingers touch. Then the hands separate, connecting again at the moon mound so that the pinky side of the hands is touching.

Repeat this movement by turning the palms out and striking the sides of the index fingers together again. When the hands connect, chant the mantra "Har" with the tip of the tongue, pulling the navel in on each repetition.

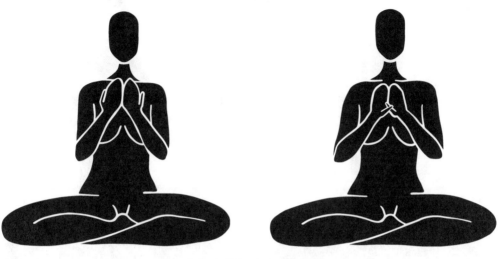

Subagh Kriya Action Part I

Repetition: The exercise is completed for three minutes.

Checking the Technique: The navel is pulled in toward the spine with each chant of "Har."

Part II

Mudra: Fingers stretch wide, actively pulling away from each other.

Drishti: The eyes close, gaze focusing on the third eye.

Mantra: "Har" is chanted internally.

Technique: Arms are stretched upward at a sixty-degree angle and the fingers are spread wide.

Action: Slightly in front of the body, the arms begin crossing one another in front of the face. The arms alternate: the right arm crosses the left, followed by the left arm crossing the right. Keep the arms straight with no bend in the elbows.

The mantra "Har" is internally chanted each time the wrists cross. The in and out motion moves at the same cadence as it did in part I.

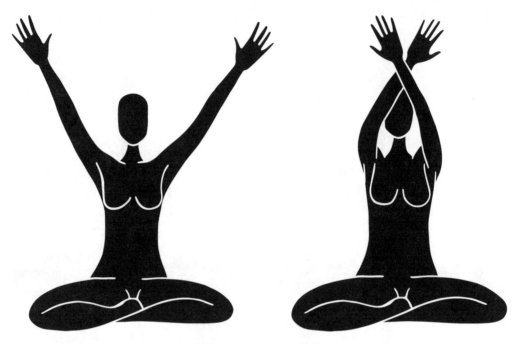

Subagh Kriya Action Part II

Repetition: The exercise is completed for three minutes. Leave the arms raised as you transition to part III.

Checking the Technique: "Har" is repeated internally at the same cadence as the previous mantra. As the arms cross, the palms remain facing forward with the arms straight and engaged.

Part III

Mudra: Each thumb crosses the palms, touching the pinky mound. The four remaining fingers wrap around the thumb, creating a fist.

Drishti: The eyes close, gaze focusing on the third eye.

Mantra: "God" is chanted externally.

Technique: The arms are outstretched at a sixty-degree angle and the thumbs are aggressively squeezed within the fists.

Action: The arms begin rotating in small, backward circles in cadence with the breath. With each completion of a circle, the word "God" is spoken out loud.

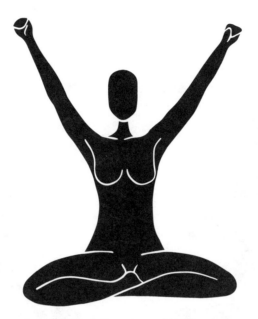

Subagh Kriya Action Part III

Repetition: The exercise is completed for three minutes.

Checking the Technique: Activate every part of your upper extremities, including your fingers, which are tightly closed around the thumbs. With the arms straight like rods, the circling will be so powerful that the entire spine will shake.

Part IV

Mudra: The palms face the body with the thumb side of the hand facing up. All fingers are pressed against one another.

Drishti: The eyes close, gaze focusing on the third eye.

Mantra: "Har Haray Haree. Wahe Guru."

Technique: The arms move up and down from the navel to the throat in a chopping motion at the same cadence as parts I, II, and III.

Action: The spine is straight and eyes are softly closed. The hands chop up and down as the mantra is chanted. To chop the hands, the left hand raises a few inches while the right hand lowers, then they reverse directions. The motion is quick and firm as your arms cut through the air.

Chant the mantra in a deep, monotonous voice for the first minute. The mantra should be repeated once every four seconds. Whisper the mantra for the second minute, then whistle at the same cadence for the third.

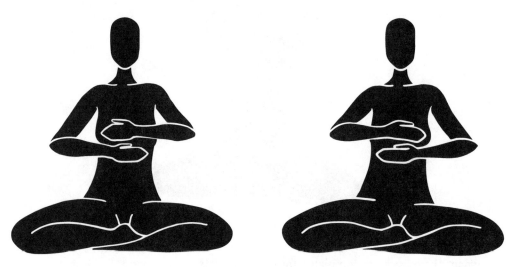

Subagh Kriya Action Part IV

Repetition: The exercise is completed for three minutes.

Checking the Technique: As you chop the hands, the arms remain engaged. Feel the biceps flex as you move.

Part V

Mudra: With both arms in front of the body, the right forearm rests on the left with the palms facing downward. The arms are in alignment with the shoulders, elevated above the heart center.

Drishti: The eyes close, gaze focusing on the third eye.

Mantra: No mantra is chanted.

Technique: Sit tall in an easy pose with the arms folded at chest height.

Action: With closed eyes, perform a one-minute breath for three minutes. This technique is physically stationary, but the inhale, retention, and exhalation of a one-minute breath create movement in the diaphragm.

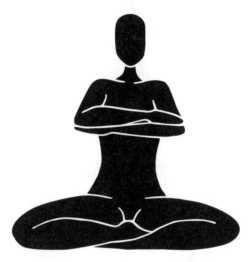

Subagh Kriya Action Part V

Repetition: The exercise is completed for three minutes.

Checking the Technique: Fill the body with air first from the abdomen, then the chest, and finally the clavicle. Hold the breath at the top of the inhalation and apply root lock, allowing the energy to circulate. On the exhale, release the air first from the clavicle, then the chest, and finally the abdomen.

Benefits: Can bring prosperity and wealth.

Conclusion

As this book comes to a close, I want to share with vulnerable honesty the conditions under which this book was written. As rock bottoms are ever so often the catalyst for change, this book began with a lifelong dream of putting pen to paper and the desire to be of service. My intention was to create a work that would help so many others, regardless of the hardship or cost endured to bring these words to life. This book's proposal was in the works when a professional rock bottom catapulted this task to the forefront of my existence. The Universe threw me out of the nest like a baby bird afraid to fly. I grew my wings as I boarded a plane to India, bowing at the feet of masters, dedicating my entirety to studying the lineage and sharing its wisdom.

The book proposal for this work was written in seven countries. My intuition guided me as I traveled through India, Greece, Austria, Croatia, Italy, France, and England, writing, growing, and hitting new highs and lows I was unaware possible. Each lesson grew more intense as I poured my heart and soul into the proposal for this manuscript. As I prepared to return to the states, I fell ill, catching a (as we say in the south) death of cold after getting caught for hours in a London rainfall. Tired and weary from months on the road, I returned back to the United States deeply ill, an illness I now believe to be COVID-19. I was in bed for over two weeks and rushed to urgent care, the sickest I can remember being in my life. In October of 2019, the pandemic was just beginning to come to the forefront of European concern—the part of the world I had just traveled across by plane, train, bus, ship, and automobile for the last four months.

As the pandemic crept onto US soil, I found myself unable to secure full-time employment, and month-by-month, even after securing a book deal, I found myself selling off my possessions one-by-one in order to pay my mortgage and keep the dream of this manuscript alive. I finally secured a verbal offer for employment out west, and just as I prepared to place my home on the market, New York City shut down. Charlotte followed shortly after. COVID-19 had reached the US, and the lockdowns of 2020 began. What was meant to be a short monthlong stay in my hometown to gain my footing and find permanent residence in California turned into an over-a-year-long struggle. The offer of full-time employment fell through as the world screeched to a halt. People were essentially locked in their homes, a catalyst that sent me into a deep and terrifying depression—a battle I came piercingly close to losing.

The month of transition in my hometown put me face-to-face with every childhood wound and heartache still torturing my soul. It was a disastrous and tumultuous year filled with heartache, pain, and the writing of this book. I lived in three different homes—four, if you count the brief interlude with a suitor—taking respite for a week at a time in eight different cities and sleeping in a total of twelve different beds and couches as the year of twists and turns continued to bob and weave. The days and nights spent penning this manuscript were some of the hardest of my life. After losing my mother to cancer and surviving a terrible divorce, miscarriages, and more than one sexual assault, I cannot fully compare one extreme to another, but I can say with all honesty that the dedication, vulnerability, and sheer tenacity required to complete this manuscript with an open heart while in the midst of immense personal pain during an unprecedented time in history will be etched in the fabric of my existence as one of my greatest hurdles and triumphs.

I tell you the story of this book's birth and the depth of my depression to bring that which might reside in the shadows into the light. There was a time during the pandemic when I saw no one for three weeks. The isolation mandated by the government, combined with the isolation of writing this book, compounded by the shame of no income and the gamble of this soul's calling, sent me into a downward spiral that I feared I may not climb out of. If it wasn't for my pup, my dear Jackson, I am relatively certain I would not be here today. It was because of his well-being and my fear for his care and safety that I finally found the strength to do whatever necessary to pull myself from the darkness. Grace be for the love of our animals, and I owe my life, and the beating of my heart, many times over to my dear Jackieboy.

I share this component of my tale for I want you to understand that you are, in fact, never alone. I almost lost myself while writing this manuscript, and yet, somehow, the book has concluded and I am able to pen these words to you today. Know that you are whole and perfect exactly as you are. Should you feel things are beyond your control, reach out to someone—anyone—who can get you the help you need: a local therapist, a counselor, a trusted friend. There are resources at your disposal and individuals who, more than anything, want you to have the opportunity to share the gift of your life, in all its grace and beauty, with the world.

You matter. Your thoughts matter. Your beliefs matter. YOU matter. Never forget that you are loved. Loved and divinely supported. My arms open wide and my heart prays for your safety and happiness. I hope that we meet someday and, on that day, I wish for nothing less than for all of your greatest dreams, hopes, and joys to be fulfilled.

Time is our most valuable asset, and I thank you for the gift of sharing it with me. I don't take this energetic exchange lightly. I pray that the contents within serve you, and will continue to serve you, all of the long days of your life.

With immense love and gratitude. Sat Nam.

Forever Your Friend
Erin

One-, Three-, and Eleven-Minute Exercises

A LIST OF TECHNIQUES by duration and where to find them.

One-Minute Exercises

Chapter Three: Shine Like a Yogi
Spinal Flexion
Spinal Twists
Sufi Grinds

Chapter Four: Balance Like a Yogi
Chandra Bhedana Pranayama (Left Nostril Breathing)
Surya Bhedana Pranayama (Right Nostril Breathing)
Nadi Shodhana Pranayama (Alternate Nostril Breathing)

Chapter Five: Nourish Like a Yogi
Stretch Pose
Frog Squats

Chapter Six: Sit Like a Yogi
Ardha Padmasana (Half Lotus)
Padmasana (Lotus)
Siddhasana (Accomplished Pose for Men)
Siddha Yoni Asana (Accomplished Pose for Women)
Vajrasana (Thunderbolt)
Shoulder Shrugs

Chapter Seven: Breathe Like a Yogi
Kapalabhati Pranayama (Skull Shining Breath)
Ujjayi Pranayama (Ocean Breath)
Sheetali Pranayama (Hissing Breath)
Sheetkari Pranayama (Hissing Breath Variation)
Bhramari Pranayama (Bee Breath)

Chapter Nine: Squeeze Like a Yogi
Moola Bandha (Root Lock)
Uddiyana Bandha (Abdomen Lock)

Jalandhara Bandha (Throat Lock)
Maha Bandha (The Great Lock)

Chapter Eleven: Practice Like a Yogi
Ego Eradicator

Three-Minute Exercises

Chapter Two: Manifest Like a Yogi
Swan Kriya
Sat Kriya

Chapter Three: Shine Like a Yogi
Root Chakra Mini Meditation

Chapter Six: Sit Like a Yogi
Meditation on the White Swan

Chapter Eight: Gesture Like a Yogi
Excel, Excel, Fearless Meditation

Chapter Nine: Squeeze Like a Yogi
Maha Bheda Mudra
Three-Minute Har

Chapter Eleven: Practice Like a Yogi
Meditation to Heal Addictions

Eleven-Minute Exercises

Chapter Two: Manifest Like a Yogi
Ambrosial Hours

Chapter Three: Shine Like a Yogi
Gyan Chakra Kriya

Chapter Four: Balance Like a Yogi
Tapping into Your Masculine Energy
Tapping into Your Feminine Energy

Chapter Eight: Gesture Like a Yogi
Guru Nanak's Treasure Meditation
Meditation to Get Rid of "Couldn't"

Chapter Ten: Sing Like a Yogi
Antar Naad Mudra Meditation
Meditation for Protection and Projection from the Heart
The Morning Call
Healing Meditation to Help Those in Need
Meditation for Elevation, Connection, and Joy
The "Last Resort" Meditation
Shabad Kriya

Chapter Eleven: Practice Like a Yogi
Kundalini Flu Bath
Magnificent Mantra
Subagh Kriya

Appendix B
Helpful Charts

CHARTS THAT SERVE AS a quick reference guide of the Kundalini teachings within.

Chapter One: Kunda What?

	Types of Traditional Yoga
1	Hatha
2	Karma
3	Bhakti
4	Ashtanga
5	Mantra
6	Nada
7	Kundalini

Chapter Two: Manifest Like a Yogi

	Lokahs	
	Sanskrit	*Location*
1	Satyam	Higher universes (higher lokahs) ↑
2	Tapah	↑
3	Janah	↑
4	Mahah	↑
5	Swah	Connected to the earth
6	Bhuvah	Connected to the earth
7	Bhoo	Connected to the earth
8	Tala	↓
9	Atala	↓
10	Vitala	↓
11	Sutala	↓
12	Mahatala	↓
13	Rasatala	↓
14	Patala	Lower universes (lower lokhas) Inside the earth ↓

Chapter Three: Shine Like a Yogi

	The Six Aspects of a Chakra
1	Color
2	Number of petals of the lotus flower
3	Yantra, or geometrical shape
4	Beeja, or seed mantra
5	Animal symbol
6	Higher or divine beings

	Sanskrit	*English*	*Color*
7	Sahasrara	Crown	Violet
6	Ajna	Third Eye	Indigo
5	Vishuddhi	Throat	Blue
4	Anahata	Heart	Green
3	Manipura	Solar Plexus	Yellow
2	Swadhisthana	Sacral	Orange
1	Mooladhara	Root	Red

Chapter Seven: Breathe Like a Yogi

Aspects of Pranayama		
Puraka (Shwasa)	Inhalation	The act of breathing air into the lungs
Rechaka (Prashwasa)	Exhalation	The act of releasing air from the lungs
Kumbhaka	Retention	The restriction of air between the inhale and exhale
Bahir Kumbhaka	External Retention	Mindful retention after exhalation
Aantir Kumbhaka	Internal Retention	Mindful retention after inhalation

Five Divisions of Prana (Air/Force)			
	Sanskrit	Location	Energy Flow
1	Prana	Lungs	Flows through the lungs, heart, and nostrils
2	Apana	Lower Abdomen	Flows from the lower abdomen to the elimination organs
3	Samana	Upper Abdomen	Flow of nutrition, which processes through the abdominal organs
4	Udana	Throat	Flows from the heart to the head to the brain
5	Vyana	Entire Body	Flows through the entire body including all limbs

Five Upa Pranas		
	Sanskrit	*English*
1	Naga	Burping
2	Koorma	Blinking
3	Krikara	Hunger/Thirst
4	Devadatta	Sneezing
5	Dhananjaya	Rigor Mortis

Pranayamas		
	Sanskrit	*English*
1	Kapalabhati Pranayama	Skull Shining Breath
2	Chandra Bhedana Pranayama	Left Nostril Breathing
3	Surya Bhedana Pranayama	Right Nostril Breathing
4	Nadi Shodhana Pranayama	Alternate Nostril Breathing
5	Ujjayi Pranayama	Ocean Breath
6	Sheetali Pranayama	Hissing Breath
7	Sheetkari Pranayama	Hissing Breath Variation
8	Bhastrika Pranayama	Bellows Breath
9	Bhramari Pranayama	Bee Breath

Chapter Eight: Gesture Like a Yogi

Five Groups of Yoga Mudras	
Hasa	Hand mudras
Mana	Head mudras
Kaya	Postural mudras
Bandha	Lock mudras
Adhara	Perineal mudras

Connect the Thumb with Intention	
Index finger to thumb for	Wisdom
Middle finger to thumb to	Overcome challenges
Ring finger to thumb for	Energy and vitality
Pinky finger to thumb for	Clear mind and communication

Fingers and the Elements			
Finger	Element	Planet(s)	Energy
Thumb	Earth	Mars	The ego
Index Finger	Ether/Space	Jupiter	Hurdles disappear
Middle Finger	Air	Saturn	Purity and piety
Ring Finger	Fire	Sun & Venus	Health
Pinky Finger	Water	Mercury	Friendship and prosperity

Hasta (Hand Mudras)	Adhara (Perineal Mudras)	Kaya (Postural Mudras)	Bandha (Lock Mudras)	Mana (Head Mudras)
Jnana Mudra	Ashwini Mudra	Viparita Karani Mudra	Maha Mudra	Shambhavi Mudra
Gyan Mudra	Vajroli/Saha-joli Mudra	Pashinee Mudra	Maha Bheda Mudra	Nasikagra Drishti Mudra
Yoni Mudra		Prana Mudra	Maha Vedha Mudra	Khechari Mudra
Bhairava Mudra		Yoga Mudra		Kaki Mudra
Hridaya Mudra		Manduki Mudra		Bhujangini Mudra
		Tadagi Mudra		Bhoochari Mudra
				Akashi Mudra
				Shanmukhi Mudra
				Unmani Mudra

Glossary

Aantir Kumbhaka: Internal retention. Mindful retention after inhalation

Adhara: Perineal mudras redirecting prana from the lower chakras to the brain. Associated with the movement of sexual energy

Agni: Ayurvedic term describing the strength of one's digestive system, or digestive fire

Ahimsa: One of the five Yamas. Nonviolence; not injuring or showing cruelty to any creature or person

Ajna: The third eye chakra

Akashi Mudra: A mana, or head mudra, utilizing the eyes, ears, nose, tongue, and lips

Ambrosial Hours: The time between 4:00 a.m. and 6:00 a.m., approximately two hours before sunrise near the equator, also known as brahmamuhurta

Anahata: The heart chakra

Antahkarana: Instrument of the mind

Aparigaha: One of the five Yamas. Non-possessiveness; life without worldly comforts such as possessions, status, and wealth. A life without material possessions rooted in the desire to pursue a path of spiritual enlightenment

Arc Line: One's aura

Asana: Posture. The third of the eight limbs of yoga

Ashtang Mantra: A mantra consisting of eight syllables

Ashwini Mudra: A perineal mudra that redirects prana from the lower chakras to the brain. Associated with the movement of sexual energy

Asteya: One of the five Yamas. Non-stealing; refraining from misappropriation and accepting bribes

Aura: Human energy field that extends outward past the physical form

Ayama: Expansion, extension

Ayurveda: The science of life

Bahir Kumbhaka: External retention. Mindful retention after exhalation

Bandha: To hold, tighten, or lock. Lock mudras are used to charge the body with prana and ignite Kundalini awakening

Beeja Mantras: Seed mantras, correlating to the seven chakras

Bhairava Mudra: A hasta, or hand mudra, used to redirect the prana emitted in the hands back into the body, generating a loop of energy between the hand and the brain

Bhastrika: Also known as Bellows Breath or Breath of Fire

Brahmacarya: One of the five Yamas. Celibacy; a state in which one is free from all sexual desires

Brahmamuhurta: The divine time. See *ambrosial hours*

Brahmari: Also known as Bee Breath

Chakra: Energy centers found within the body that run from the base of the spine to the crown of the head

Chandra Bhedana Pranayama: Also known as Left Nostril Breathing

Chin Mudra: See *Gyan Mudra*

Devadatta: Sneezing; cleansing of the nose and sinuses. One of the five upa pranas

Dhananjaya: Rigor mortis; leaving the body after death. One of the five upa pranas

Dharana: Concentration and focus. The sixth of the eight limbs of yoga

Dharma: An individual's duty fulfilled in observance of Cosmic Law, including duties, rights, laws, conduct, virtues, and the "right" way of living

Dhyana: Meditation. The seventh of the eight limbs of yoga

Drishti: Focused gaze

Exhalation: The act of releasing air from the lungs

External Retention: Mindful holding of one's breath after exhalation

Granthi: Knot, doubt

Gyan Mudra: A hasta, or hand mudra, used to redirect the prana emitted in the hands back into the body, generating a loop of energy between the hand and the brain. Also known as Chin Mudra

Hasta: Hand mudra. Used predominantly in meditation to redirect the prana emitted in the hands back into the body, generating a loop of energy between the hand and the brain

Hridaya Mudra: A hasta, or hand mudra, used to redirect the prana emitted in the hands back into the body, generating a loop of energy between the hand and the brain

Ida: The nadi associated with the left hemisphere of the body. Feminine energy

Inhalation: The act of breathing air into the lungs

Internal Retention: Mindful retention after inhalation

Jnana Mudra: A hasta, or hand mudra, used to redirect the prana emitted in the hands back into the body, generating a loop of energy between the hand and the brain

Jupiter: The side of the hand along the index finger. See *moon mound*

Kaki Mudra: A mana, or head mudra, utilizing the eyes, ears, nose, tongue, and lips

Kapalbhati: Also known as Skull Shining Breath

Karma: A person's destiny, or fate, created by the sum of their actions in past lives and their current incarnation

Kaya: Postural mudras combining breath work, physical postures, and mental concentration

Khechari Mudra: A mana, or head mudra, utilizing the eyes, ears, nose, tongue, and lips

Koorma: Blinking; cleansing of the eyes. One of the five upa pranas

Kridayakasha: The space within the heart where purity resides

Krikara: Hunger/thirst. One of the five upa pranas

Kriya: A technique or practice executed to achieve a particular result

Kumbhaka: See *retention*

Kundalini: The yogic life force that is said to lie dormant. When the body is unblocked and the chakras are aligned, one's Kundalini energy can be awakened, making its way up the body toward enlightenment

Kundalini Energy: Represented by a snake coiled three and a half times. Located behind the mooladhara chakra at the base of the spine

Kurma: See *koorma*

Lokah: The fourteen universes, per the Vedic scriptures

Long Time Sun: A closing prayer. Typically sung at the end of each Kundalini class in the Yogi Bhajan tradition

Mahakala: Great or endless time. The Kundalini serpent

Mana: A head mudra utilizing the eyes, ears, nose, tongue, and lips; an integral part of the practice of Kundalini yoga

Manipura: The solar plexus chakra

Mantra: A word or sound repeated. Assists with concentration in meditation

Mauna: Complete silence

Mooladhara: The root chakra

Moon Mound: The side of the hand along the pinky finger. See *Jupiter*

Mudra: A gesture or attitude

Nadis: More than 72,000 energy channels located throughout the body

Nadi Shodhana Pranayama: Also known as Alternate Nostril Breathing

Naga: Burping. One of the five upa pranas

Nasikagra Drishti: A mana, or head mudra, utilizing the eyes, ears, nose, tongue, and lips

Niyama: Fixed observance, regularity, and self-purification. The second of the eight limbs of yoga

Ong Namo Guru Dev Namo: Mantra traditionally used to begin a Kundalini class in the Yogi Bhajan tradition. It means "I bow to the creative wisdom. I bow to the divine teacher within"

Pashinee Mudra: A kaya, or postural mudra, that combines breath work, physical posture, and mental concentration

Perineum: The location of the mooladhara chakra, midway between the genitals and anus

Pingala: The nadi associated with the right hemisphere of the body. Masculine energy

Pooraka: See *inhalation*

Prajna: Intuition

Prana: Breath; life force energy

Prana Mudra: A kaya, or postural mudra, that combines breath work, physical posture, and mental concentration

Pranayama: Breath control. The fourth of the eight limbs of yoga

Pranotthana: Pranic force

Prarabdha Karma: Destiny, fate

Pratyahara: The withdrawal of the senses. The fifth of the eight limbs of yoga

Puraka (Shwasa): An alternate spelling of *pooraka*

Rajas: A tendency toward passion, ambition, and assertiveness

Raniki: The goddess of the vegetable kingdom

Rechaka (Prashwasa): See *exhalation*

Retention: The restriction of air in the space between an inhale and exhale; the pause between breaths

Sadhana: The act of a daily practice. A daily dedication to one's spiritual practice

Sahajoli/Vajroli Mudra: A perineal mudra that redirects prana from the lower chakras. Associated with the movement of sexual energy

Sahasrara: The crown chakra

Samadhi: Salvation or super-consciousness. The eighth and final limb of the eight limbs of yoga

Sat Nam: Mantra traditionally used to close a Kundalini class in the Yogi Bhajan tradition. A beeja or seed mantra that means "Truth is my identity. I am truth"

Satya: One of the five Yamas. To speak the truth; including the consideration of what is said, as well as how it is said, and how it could affect others

Seed Mantra: See *beeja mantras*

Shakti: The divine feminine

Sheetkari Pranayama: Also known as Hissing Breath Variation

Sheetali Pranayama: Also known as Hissing Breath

Shiva: The divine masculine

Shoonya: Void. Often described as what one sees when the eyes are closed and the drishti is focused on the third eye

Shuniaa: An alternate spelling of *Shoonya*

Solmization: Assigning syllables to steps of the musical scale

Surya Bhedana Pranayama: Also known as Right Nostril Breathing

Sushumna: The central nadi running from the base of the spine through the crown of the head. The nadi where all other nadis intersect. Associated with the balance between masculine and feminine energy

Swadhisthana: The sacral chakra

Tadagi Mudra: A kaya, or postural mudra, that combines breath work, physical posture, and mental concentration

Tapas: The vigor and intensity of the efforts of performing a spiritual discipline

Ujjayi Pranayama: Also known as Ocean Breath

Unmani Mudra: A mana, or head mudra, utilizing the eyes, ears, nose, tongue, and lips

Upa Prana: Minor pranas consisting of burping, blinking, hunger/thirst, sneezing, and rigor mortis

Vajroli/Sahajoli Mudra: A perineal mudra that redirects prana from the lower chakras. Associated with the movement of sexual energy

Vedas: The oldest writings of Hinduism filled with verses, or mantras

Viparita Karani Mudra: A kaya, or postural mudra, that combines breath work, physical posture, and mental concentration

Vipasyana: Special seeing or insight. Alternate spelling of Vipassana in the West. One of India's most sacred techniques of meditation

Vishnu Granthi: The second psychic knot, located at the anahata

Vishuddhi: The throat chakra

Yama: Control. The first of the eight limbs of yoga. Moral discipilines and vows

Yantra: The third element of a chakra, its geometric shape. This world can also refer to a mystical diagram used as a meditative tool

Yoga Mudra: A kaya, or postural mudra, that combines breath work, physical posture, and mental concentration

Yogic Breath: Controlled breathing in three parts: first filling the abdomen with air, then the chest, and finally the clavicle. The exhale of the breath is also in three parts, beginning with the clavicle and ending with the abdomen

Yoni Mudra: A hasta, or hand mudra, used to redirect the prana emitted in the hands back into the body, generating a loop of energy between the hand and the brain

Recommended Reading

IF YOU'D LIKE TO learn more about the different lineages of Kundalini yoga, including Kundalini yoga as taught by Yogi Bhajan, there are plenty of excellent resources. This recommended reading list is not meant to be comprehensive; it is only a starting point for your continued learning.

Singh Khalsa, Nirvair. *The Art, Science & Application of Kundalini Yoga*. 4th ed. Santa Cruz, NM: Kundalini Research Institute, 2015.

Yogi Bhajan. *Infinity and Me: Kundalini Yoga as Taught by Yogi Bhajan*. Santa Cruz, NM: Kundalini Research Institute, 2004.

Yogi Bhajan and Harijot Kaur Khalsa. *Owner's Manual for the Human Body: Kundalini Yoga as Taught by Yogi Bhajan*. Santa Cruz, NM: Kundalini Research Institute, 1993.

———. *Physical Wisdom: Kundalini Yoga as Taught by Yogi Bhajan*. Santa Cruz, NM: Kundalini Research Institute, 1994.

———. *Reaching ME in Me: Kundalini Yoga as Taught by Yogi Bhajan*. Santa Cruz, NM: Kundalini Research Institute, 2000.

———. *Self-Experience: Kundalini Yoga as Taught by Yogi Bhajan*. Santa Cruz, NM: Kundalini Research Institute, 2000.

———. *Self-Knowledge: Kundalini Yoga as Taught by Yogi Bhajan*. Santa Cruz, NM: Kundalini Research Institute, 1995.

Bibliography

Adams, Mitzi, Beth Bero, and Tom Sever. "Planetarium Program" in *The Sun in Time*. NASA. Accessed March 9, 2021. https://solarscience.msfc.nasa.gov/suntime/talk2 .stm.

Admin. "Forward Head Posture / 'Text Neck Syndrome.'" Health Blog. Greenhaus Physical Therapy, January 15, 2016. https://www.greenhauspt.com/the-quest-for-zero -infections-a-fools-mission-3/.

Asprey, Dave. "Health Benefits of Red Light Therapy and How to Get It." *Dave Asprey* (blog). Accessed March 9. 2021. https://daveasprey.com/health-benefits-red-light -therapy/.

Beirne, Geraldine. "Yoga: A Beginner's Guide to the Different Styles." *The Guardian*, January 10, 2014. https://www.theguardian.com/lifeandstyle/2014/jan/10/yoga -beginners-guide-different-styles.

Bishop, Jordan. "How to Beat Jet Lag Once and for All." *Forbes*, November 28, 2016. https://www.forbes.com/sites/bishopjordan/2016/11/28/how-to-beat-jet-lag/.

Cherry, Kendra. "The Color Psychology of White." *Verywell Mind*. Updated January 17, 2020. https://www.verywellmind.com/color-psychology-white-2795822.

Chislett, David. "What Are the Oldest Languages on Earth?" Taleninstituut Nederland, November 14, 2016. https://taleninstituut.nl/what-are-the-oldest-languages-on -earth/.

Cronkleton, Emily. "What Are the Benefits of a Baking Soda Bath, How Do You Take One, and Is It Safe?" *Healthline*. Updated September 18, 2018. https://www.healthline .com/health/baking-soda-bath.

Daily Meditate. "Meditation Quote 3: 'You Should Sit in Meditation for Twenty Minutes Every Day—Unless You're Too Busy; Then You Should Sit for an Hour.' –Zen Proverb." April 11, 2014. https://dailymeditate.com/meditation-quote-3-you-should-sit-in-meditation-for-twenty-minutes-every-day-unless-youre-too-busy-then-you-should-sit-for-an-hour-zen-proverb/.

Devika. "8 Reasons Why Eating with Hands Is Awesome." *Spoon University* (blog), *Her Campus*. Accessed March 11, 2021. https://spoonuniversity.com/lifestyle/8-reasons-eating-hands-awesome.

"Feng Shui Use of Crystal Bowls." The Spruce. Updated August 2, 2019. https://www.thespruce.com/feng-shui-use-of-crystal-bowls-1274356.

Fitzgerald, F. Scott. "The Crack-Up." *Esquire*. Last modified March 7, 2017. https://www.esquire.com/lifestyle/a4310/the-crack-up/.

Frothingham, Scott. "What Is Expiratory Reserve Volume and How Is It Measured?" *Healthline*. Updated October 19, 2018. https://www.healthline.com/health/expiratory-reserve-volume.

"Gas and Bloating." Turkish Airlines. Accessed March 9, 2021. https://www.turkishairlines.com/en-us/flights/fly-different/fly-good-feel-good/after-flight/gas-and-swelling/.

Grant, Steve. "Flying Considerations: Effects of Air Cabin Pressure on Digestion." *Steve Grant Health* (blog). Accessed March 11, 2021. https://www.stevegranthealth.com/articles/flying-considerations-effects-air-cabin-pressure-digestion/.

"The Granthis." Sheshnaag Yoga Centre. Accessed March 15, 2021. https://www.sheshnaag.com/the-granthis/.

Healthline Wellness Team. "Infrared Saunas: Your Questions Answered." *Healthline*. Updated April 10, 2019. https://www.healthline.com/health/under-review-infrared-saunas.

Helmenstine, Anne Marie. "How Long You Can Live Without Food, Water, or Sleep." ThoughtCo. Updated August 8, 2019. https://www.thoughtco.com/living-without-food-water-sleep-4138375.

"Hot 100 Turns 60." *Billboard*, August 4, 2018. https://www.billboard.com/charts/hot-100-60th-anniversary.

"How Many Breaths You Take Per Day and Why It Matters." Advent. Accessed March 12, 2021. https://adventknows.com/blog/how-many-breaths-you-take-per-day-why-it-matters/.

"How Tibetan Singing Bowls Affect Our Body?" Hoteli Bernardin, December 11, 2018. https://www.hoteli-bernardin.si/en/blog/wellness/2334-How-Tibetan-singing -bowls-affect-our-body.

Ishwardas Chunilal Yogic Health Center. *Prayer and Mantrajapa*. Maharashtra, India: Kaivalyadhama, n.d.

Jain, Mayank. "Ban on Cow Slaughter in 24 Indian States Is Leading to Dead Humans on the Border." *Scroll*, November 11, 2014. https://scroll.in/article/689155/Ban-on -cow-slaughter-in-24-Indian-states-is-leading-to-dead-humans-on-the-border.

Johnston, Cassie. "Sprouting 101: How to Sprout Anything and Why You Should." Wholefully. Accessed March 11, 2021. https://wholefully.com/sprouting-101/.

Kaur Khalsa, Siri-Ved. *From Vegetables, With Love: Recipes & Tales from a Yogi's Kitchen*. Santa Cruz, NM: Kundalini Research Institute, 2015.

Korenic, Eileen, and Joseph Shaw. "Why Is the Sky Blue? Why Are Sunsets Red?" Optics for Kids. Accessed March 9, 2021. https://www.optics4kids.org/what-is -optics/scattering/why-is-the-sky-blue-why-are-sunsets-red.

Kovalchik, Kara. "Why Are Notes of the Tonal Scale Called 'Do, Re, Mi' etc.?" *Mental Floss*, October 28, 2013. https://www.mentalfloss.com/article/53280/why-are-notes -tonal-scale-called-do-re-mi.

"Kundalini Yoga Mantras." 3HO. Accessed March 16, 2021. https://www.3ho.org /kundalini-yoga/mantra/kundalini-yoga-mantras.

"The Mantra Toolkit: Ad Guray Nameh." 3HO. Accessed March 16, 2021. https:// www.3ho.org/kundalini-yoga/mantra/kundalini-yoga-mantras/mantra-toolkit -ad-guray-nameh.

"The Mantra Toolkit: Har Har Har Har Gobinday." 3HO. Accessed March 16, 2021. https://www.3ho.org/kundalini-yoga/mantra/kundalini-yoga-mantras/mantra -toolkit-har-har-har-har-gobinday.

Mayo Clinic Staff. "Water: How Much Should You Drink Every Day?" Mayo Clinic Healthy Lifestyle, Nutrition and Healthy Eating. October 14, 2020. https://www .mayoclinic.org/healthy-lifestyle/nutrition-and-healthy-eating/in-depth/water/art -20044256.

Mead, M. Nathaniel. "Benefits of Sunlight: A Bright Spot for Human Health." *Environmental Health Perspective* 116, no. 4 (April 2008): A160–67. https://doi.org/10.1289 /ehp.116-a160.

"Meditation for Elevation, Connection, and Joy." 3HO. Accessed March 16, 2021. https://www.3ho.org/kundalini-yoga/chakras/meditation-elevation-connection -and-joy.

Myers, Amy. "6 Benefits of Infrared Sauna Therapy." Amy Myers MD. Updated February 24, 2021. https://www.amymyersmd.com/article/benefits-infrared-sauna -therapy/.

Parwha Kaur Khalsa, Shakti. "My Favorite Mantra: Ek Ong Kar Sat Nam Siri Wahe Guru." 3HO. Accessed March 16, 2021. https://www.3ho.org/kundalini-yoga /meditation/featured-meditations/my-favorite-mantra-ek-ong-kar-sat-nam -siri-wahe-guru.

Physiopedia Contributors. "Forward Head Posture." *Physiopedia*. Updated April 28, 2020. https://www.physio-pedia.com/Forward_Head_Posture.

Pilates, Joseph H., and William John Miller. *Return to Life Through Contrology*. New York: J. J. Augustin, 1945.

"Principles of Yoga—3 Granthis." Sanjeeva Ayurveda Wellness Center at Vedic Village. Accessed March 15, 2021. http://www.sanjeeva.net/the-3granthis.html.

Ramos, Juan. "What Continent Is India in?" Science Trends, January 5, 2018. https:// sciencetrends.com/heres-continent-india/.

"Red Light Therapy Benefits & How It Works." Joovv, updated June 28, 2021. https:// joovv.com/blogs/joovv-blog/how-does-red-light-therapy-work.

Saeed, Sadia. "Mindfulness Is Untying the Knots." Mindful Spring, September 25, 2017. http://mindfulspring.com/mindfulness-untying-knots-buddha-story/.

Saradananda, Swami. *Mudras for Modern Life: Boost Your Health, Enhance Your Yoga and Deepen Your Meditation*. London: Watkins, 2015.

Satyananda Saraswati, Swami. *Asana Pranayama Mudra Bandha*. Munger, Bihar, India: Yoga Publications Trust, 2013.

———. *Kundalini Tantra*. Munger, Bihar, India: Yoga Publications Trust, 2013.

———. *Mudra Vigyan: Philosophy and Practice of Yogic Gestures*. Munger, Bihar, India: Yoga Publications Trust, 2013.

Scott, Christopher K. "Life's Currency: ATP." In *A Primer for the Exercise and Nutrition Sciences*. Totowa, NJ: Humana Press, 2008. https://doi.org/10.1007/978-1-60327 -383-1_8.

Sikhnet. "Yogi Bhajan." The Sikh Network, 2004. http://fateh.sikhnet.com/yogibhajan.

"Silver Gallery." Museo de Arte Precolombino (Museum of Pre-Columbian Art). Accessed March 9, 2021. https://mapcusco.pe/en/salas/silver/.

Singh Sahib, Siri. *Success and the Spirit: An Aquarian Path to Abundance*. Española, NM: Sikh Dharma International, 2011.

Spritzler, Franziska. "10 Evidence-Based Health Benefits of Magnesium." *Healthline*, September 3, 2018. https://www.healthline.com/nutrition/10-proven-magnesium -benefits.

Sterbenz, Christina. "12 Famous Quotes that Always Get Misattributed." *Insider*, October 7, 2013. https://www.businessinsider.com/misattributed-quotes-2013-10.

Suni, Eric. "Melatonin and Sleep." Sleep Foundation. Updated August 6, 2020. https:// www.sleepfoundation.org/melatonin.

Tello, Monique. "Intermittent Fasting: Surprising Update." Harvard Health Publishing. Updated February 10, 2020. https://www.health.harvard.edu/blog/intermittent -fasting-surprising-update-2018062914156.

The Teachings of Yogi Bhajan. "Yogi Bhajan's Words on Wearing White." 3HO. Accessed March 3, 2021. https://www.3ho.org/ecommunity/2012/11/yogi-bhajans -words-on-wearing-white.

Tripp, Megan. "Hot Yoga vs Bikram Yoga: What's the Difference?" *Boston Magazine*, September 11, 2013. https://www.bostonmagazine.com/health/2013/09/11/what-is -the-difference-between-hot-yoga-and-bikram-yoga/.

Victoria State Government Department of Health. "Digestive System Explained." Better Health Channel. Reviewed August 31, 2014. https://www.betterhealth.vic.gov.au /health/conditionsandtreatments/digestive-system.

"The Water in You: Water and the Human Body." USGS. Accessed March 9, 2021. https://www.usgs.gov/special-topic/water-science-school/science/water-you-water -and-human-body?qt-science_center_objects=0#qt-science_center_objects.

Winston, Kimberly. "The 'Splainer: What Makes the Cow Sacred to Hindus?" *The Washington Post*, November 5, 2015. https://www.washingtonpost.com/national /religion/the-splainer-what-makes-the-cow-sacred-to-hindus/2015/11/05 /acdde3e2-840c-11e5-8bd2-680fff868306_story.html.

Zimmerman, Edith. "What Is Autophagy?" *The Cut*, April 25, 2019. https://www .thecut.com/2019/04/what-is-autophagy.html.